# COPYRIGHT

No part of this book may be produced, reproduced, stored in any retrieval system or transmitted in any form or any means, electronic, mechanical, photocopying, recording or otherwise without prior permission from the author or Amazon's create space on that behalf

I0790835

## APPRECIATION

The author acknowledges the continued support from daughters Mercy and Monica; Niece Julia and Ken Kinoti

# PREFACE

Diabetes mellitus (DM) has been labeled the epidemic of the 21st century, claiming its toll on both quality and duration of life and posing a major economic burden to society. By the year 2050, it is predicted that one in every ten people (10%) in the population will be diagnosed with DM. This is against a background of remarkable progress in data collection and information dissemination regarding the disease. This implies that more still needs to be done in terms of information sharing. According to the American Diabetes Association (ADA), United States alone had nearly 7 million undiagnosed cases of diabetes by the time of writing this book (2017). This could be attributed to the fact that early symptoms of diabetes, especially type 2 diabetes are not a direct indication of a disease and may appear seemingly harmless. However, once the condition establishes itself, it causes untold suffering; for example in the industrialized countries, diabetes is the second cause of blindness, third cause of renal failure, is responsible for half of the amputations of lower limbs and is one of the primary causes of death  Whereas in yester years there was scarcity of information, the world is currently engulfed in a sea of facts but getting what you need in one piece might take a very long time and you might end up frustrated and without the much needed information.  This book packages diabetes information in form of a real practical account of type 2 diabetes. It examines the pre and post diagnosis of the disease and it tries to give a scientific justification on the signs that were experienced during that period. In compiling this book, a lot of data was collected and analyzed over time on factors such as blood pressure, weight, exercise and so on; however the information that was given preference in the book was in regard to non-medical control of diabetes especially through lifestyle change.

During the observation period, 6 key factors were found to contribute significantly to the control of the blood sugars. These are; early detection, type of food, method of food preparation, regularity in spacing the meals, exercise and record keeping on important parameters such as weight, blood pressure and blood sugar levels. From the onset, the author took risks by making fewer consultations with a medical practitioner and a nutritionist, factors that might have contributed to the long time (two years) taken to control the sugars. The experimental nature of this work is not encouraged to patients as the author who is a veterinarian had some scientific information on the disease in animals and which she used frequently to compare with her situation.

This book is the first in a series that will be used to update the reader on the control progress. The book is recommended for people who do not have much training on the disease due to the simplicity of the compiled literature in the body of the report, which is the first part. It could also be of interest to scholars due to the attached data in form of annexes.

# TABLE OF CONTENTS


COPYRIGHT ........................................................................................................................ i

APPRECIATION ............................................................................................................... ii

PREFACE ............................................................................................................................ iii

TABLE OF CONTENTS .................................................................................................. iv

LIST OF TABLES .............................................................................................................. v

LIST OF FIGURES ........................................................................................................... vi

1. PRE-DIABETES DIAGNOSIS ................................................................................... 1

   1.1 Background information ........................................................................................... 1

   1.2 Clinical signs and how I had managed them before the diabetes diagnosis ............ 1

      1.2.1 Left foot lesions ............................................................................................... 1

      1.2.2 Fleeting increased heart beat (tachycardia) .................................................... 2

      1.2.3 Excessive thirst ............................................................................................... 4

      1.2.4 Polycystic ovary syndrome (PCOS) ............................................................... 4

      1.2.5 Other predisposing factors .............................................................................. 5

2. POST DIABETES DIAGNOSIS .................................................................................. 7

   2.1: Stage 1(May -June 2014) - Intense Injectable and Non-Injectable Medication ..... 7

   2.2: Stage 2(July -December 2014): Non-injectable medication ................................. 11

   2.3: Stage 3: January-May 2015: Diet takes Center stage ......................................... 13

   2.4: Stage 4(June -December 2015)- No Diabetic medication , Glycemic Index above 6mmol/l .......... 16

   2.5 Stage 5(January to May 2016): No medication – GI less than 6mmol/l ................ 17

3. LESSONS LEARNT ...................................................................................................... 19

4. ANNEXES .................................................................................................................... 21

   Annex 1: Data on Stage 1(May 2014-June 2014) - Intense Injectable and Non-Injectable Medication. 21

   Annex 2: Data on Stage 2(July -December 2014): Non-injectable medication ......... 22

   Annex 3: Data on Stage 3(January-May 2015: Diet takes Center stage ................... 24

   Annex 4: Data on Stage 4(June -December 2015) - No diabetes medication, Glycemic Index above 6mmol/l ......................................................................................... 29

   Annex 5- Stage 5(January to May 2016): No diabetes medication – GI less than 6mmol/l ................... 36

   Annex 6: Some common food and simple methods used to prepare them ................. 41

   Annex 7: Oat's toasted bread's breakfast ................................................................. 44

REFERENCES .................................................................................................................. 45

# LIST OF TABLES

Table 1: Laboratory results of blood analysis in January 2016 .................................................................. 18

# LIST OF FIGURES


Figure 1: Eruptive xanthomas (Duff et al, 2015)[1] ............................................................... 2
Figure 2: Blood glucose meter and related accessories ....................................................... 8
Figure 3: Digital blood pressure monitor for the wrist ....................................................... 10
Figure 4: The bathroom weighing scale ............................................................................... 13
Figure 5: Thorny melon-Not ripe (T) and ripe (B) ............................................................. 15
Figure 6: White Supote Tree (L) and Branch with Fruits (R) ............................................ 16
Figure 7: Author-Before diagnosis (L) and 2 years post diagnosis .................................... 20

# 1. PRE-DIABETES DIAGNOSIS

## 1.1 Background information

When I was diagnosed with diabetes mellitus in April 2014, it did not come as a shock, not because we have a family history of diabetes or because I had seen it coming, but because for the whole of that week, I had been experiencing polyuria and polydipsia (frequent urination and increased thirst) clinical manifestation of diabetes and therefore I was almost sure it was the case. As the week progressed I felt weaker and weaker but because I was far from home where my hospital is, I thought I would wait until the end of the week when I was due back home. By Friday, it was obvious that if I did not take myself to hospital, then I would end up being taken by well-wishers. I therefore requested a colleague who was attending the same workshop with me to take me to hospital, which he did. After the preliminary examination, the Doctor confirmed my worst fears, that I was actually suffering from type 2 diabetes mellitus (DM2) and then she went ahead and admitted me for more examinations and medical care. Throughout the week that I was in hospital, I was in denial. It can't be diabetes for real, okay I know I am overweight yes, I overeat yes, I am stressed yes, I am in the age bracket that is vulnerable to diabetes yes, but my siblings have all those characteristics and they don't have diabetes. After all diabetes has a slow onset and mine just came on suddenly within one week. It was only when I was discharged from the hospital that I took stock of my diabetes history and I realized that the signs had been there but I did not associate them with the a disease let alone diabetes.

I had chronologically had the following signs ; unexplained left foot lesions of small papules (red pimples like spots/bumps) which did not have pus, excess scaling of the left foot, a fleeting increased heart beat on days that I consumed excess food/salt, excess thirst and a momentary dizziness about once a month. These signs had been there for 3 months prior to the diagnoses. In the week prior to the detection, I had lost appetite, experienced tiredness, transient numbness of the fingers and toes. But what made me decide that enough was enough and I must go to the hospital was the feeling that I was going to faint. In addition to the clinical signs, I had diabetes predisposing factors which I had not considered before, these include being overweight, stressed, over 45 years of age, solitary life, cystic ovary removal, overworking and limited exercise. I only reflected on this signs after the Doctor sought to know if I had previously experienced any symptoms of the condition. Of course I said no but according to her; this could not be true as detailed examinations had shown that my Glycosylated hemoglobin ($HbA_{1c}$) was 11.2%, far beyond the desired less than 6.5. The $HBA_{1c}$ assists in assessing the levels of glucose in the blood during the previous 6-8 weeks.

## 1.2 Clinical signs and how I had managed them before the diabetes diagnosis

### 1.2.1 Left foot lesions

Cutaneous (skin) manifestations of systemic (generalized in the body) diseases or can be an early warning sign or a late manifestation of chronic disease. I can't exactly remember how long I had had the foot lesions but it was definitely more than one year. Only the left foot was affected and there were small papules (pimples without pus) spread on the under, side and top of the foot. The skin surrounding each pimply swelling would then scale off. Before scaling, the symptoms would resemble a condition known as Eruptive xanthomas (EX). As described by Duff[1] and others in the American Diabetes Association journal (ADA), the EX has as sudden onset of crops of yellow papules with an erythematous (reddish as with more blood) base presenting themselves on the buttocks, elbows, and knees. EX is rare and occurs more often in patients with poorly controlled type 2 diabetes. The difference between my case and these signs was that mine were on the foot. These signs would go away for some time and they would then come back. Since they were neither painful nor itchy, I would ignore them but intensify feet hygiene that include nail and skin care. However, according to mayo clinical internal medicine review, this could have been a case of poorly controlled diabetes that leads to extreme increase in triglycerides level which could be as a result of acquired defects in fat metabolism brought about by interaction of aging, weight gain, poor diet, sedentary life styles and genetic predisposition.

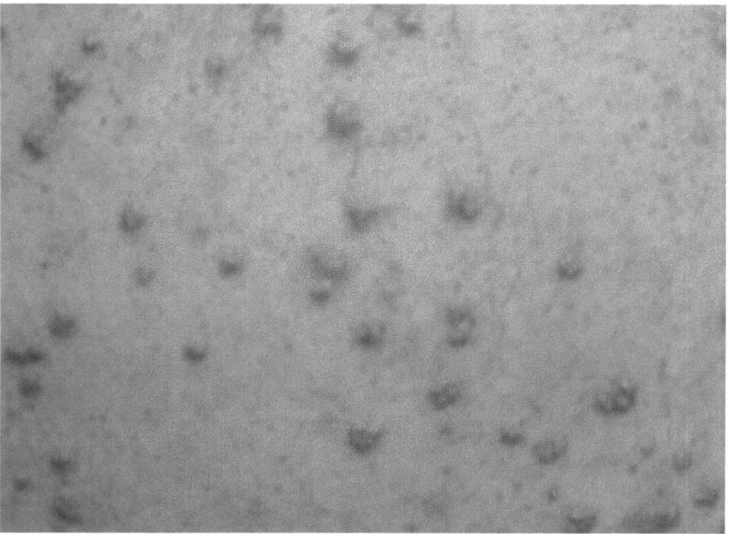

Figure 1: Eruptive xanthomas (Duff et al, 2015)[1]

1.2.2 Fleeting increased heart beat (tachycardia)
This condition was experienced mostly on Sunday afternoons. This is because Sunday is a free day and I therefore took time to enjoy my meals. I usually ate my favorite foods especially mashed food with fried beef as a side plate or other nutritious foods like chapati with rich animal protein stews. The food was always prepared the previous day as it takes a long time to cook. This means that on Sunday the food had to be heated up. The method used to do so was to fry the mash in a pan using cooking fat and onions and the tendency to add salt whether the one of the previous day was adequate or not was high. Thereafter, I used to take a nap for 2-3 hours. Three things here predisposed me to diabetes: eating foods rich in carbohydrates as the mash itself is made of very nutritious food ingredients that include maize, different types of beans, Irish potatoes and green and ripe bananas; overeating and a lot of cooking fats. Whatever food that was eaten on Sundays was high in carbohydrates.

Different carbohydrates influence the level of blood sugar immediately after the consumption a condition referred to as postprandial glycemia (glycemic index). Fiber rich foods usually have a low glycemic index (GI), although not all foods with a low GI automatically have high fiber content. Several beneficial effects of low-GI, high-fiber diets have been shown, including lower postprandial glucose and insulin responses, an improved lipid profile, and, possibly, reduced insulin resistance. The mash foods include ingredients with low fiber content and thus high GI.

The excess eating on the other hand introduces the Glycemic load (GL). This is the GI of a specific food multiplied by the amount of carbohydrate contained in an average portion of the food consumed. As described in a 2002 American journal of clinical nutrition[2], each unit of dietary GL represents the equivalent glycemic effect of 1 g carbohydrate from white bread; which is used as the reference food. As stated in a 2008 American journal of clinical nutrition[3]; in non-diabetic persons, suggestive evidence is available from epidemiological studies that a diet based on carbohydrate-rich foods with a low-GI and high-fiber content may protect against diabetes or cardiovascular disease.

Use of excess cooking fats and foods rich in animal fat introduces lipids which are basically the fats in the body which include cholesterol, triglycerides and phospholipids. Lipids are fats that are either absorbed from food or synthesized by the liver. Triglycerides (TGs) and cholesterol contribute most to disease; however, all lipids are important for the normal functions of a living thing. The primary function of TGs is to store energy in fat and muscle cells; cholesterol is a universal constituent of cell membranes, steroids and bile acids. The main components of the lipids are fatty acids which are released when the lipids are broken down. Fatty acids are absorbed through the intestine and are taken up via the lymphatic system. Fats can be utilized for energy or may be stored as adipose (fatty) tissue. All lipids are hydrophobic (not attracted to water) and mostly insoluble in blood, so they require transport within hydrophilic (attracted to water), spherical structures called lipoproteins. Lipoproteins are classified by size and density (defined as the ratio of lipid to protein) and are important because high levels of low-density lipoproteins (LDL) and low levels of high-density lipoproteins (HDL) are major risk factors for atherosclerotic (arterial blood vessel) heart disease. Animal fats are some of the common sources of LDL while plant fats are the origins of the HDL. My excess consumption of animal fats thus predisposed me to not only to obesity but also diabetes, hypertension (high blood pressure) and tachycardia (rapid heart rate). Further, it has been shown that high levels of serum/blood triglycerides or uncontrolled diabetes mellitus generally cause eruptive xanthomas and this could as well explain the foot lesions.

The increase in intensity of the heart beats could have been due to a number of other factors. Scientifically, the intestines require a large amount of blood for digestion. When blood flows to the intestines after a meal, the heart rate increases (tachycardia) and blood vessels in other parts of the body constrict to help maintain blood pressure.

Studies like that in a British Medical Journal (BMJ) of 1996[4] have shown that dietary sodium intake is positively correlated with blood pressure levels in the general population. This means that the extra salt too predisposed me to the tachycardia that was experienced after addition of salt to food. In addition to all that, the heart is a pump and the blood vessels are the pipes that the blood passes through, a high concentration of dissolved particles like glucose, table salt (sodium chloride), triglycerides and others thicken the blood and thus the heart has to mechanically exert more force and speed to deliver the blood to the normal sites. The increased heart beats used to take place during the nap and then would disappear and at that time I thought it was the overeating that caused the raised heart beats and therefore never sought medical attention. However, a combination of the factors discussed above could have been the course.

1.2.3 Excessive thirst
As early as 3 months before the diagnosis of the disease, I used to experience extreme thirst right from morning when I woke up to late in the evening when I was going to sleep. However, the thirst did not translate to increased urination probably due to the method used to quench it. Very cold consumables like ice cream or ice cubes were used to reduce the desire for a cold liquid substance. During a normal day I could consume as many as 3 ice creams and in the evening I could take several ice cubes directly from the fridge. I however did not wake up at night to quench the thirst or to urinate.

When one has diabetes, excess sugar (glucose) builds up in the blood. The kidneys are forced to work overtime to filter and absorb the excess sugar. If one's kidneys can't keep up, the excess sugar is excreted into the urine along with fluids drawn from body tissues. This triggers more frequent urination, which may leave one dehydrated. As one drinks more fluids to quench the thirst, the person will urinate even more. According to Elizabeth Furldell[5], diabetic thirst used to be fatal before introduction of Insulin. Overconsumption of table salt could also have contributed to the additional need for water. Salt provides the body with vital mineral sodium and helps maintain blood pressure and normal function of muscle and nerves. However, it is recommended that salt be used sparingly as sodium has been associated with high risk onset of blood pressure. Further, salt is a de-hydrant as it absolves water and therefore too much of it could draw fluids from the body tissues thus creating a sense of dehydration (thirst).

1.2.4 Polycystic ovary syndrome (PCOS)
According to Patient information from the BMJ Group[6] PCOS are small, fluid-filled swellings (cysts) on the ovaries. Polycystic means with lots of cysts. Doctors don't know why some women get PCOS. But it seems to run in families. One is more likely to get it if her mother had it. If one is diagnosed with polycystic ovary syndrome (PCOS) it means that her hormones are not in balance. The three types of hormones made by the ovaries are the ones most affected. They are called estrogens, androgens, and progesterone. These hormones affect a lot of things that go on in one's body, including when to have periods, when the ovaries release eggs, how hair grows on the face and body, and the condition of the skin. In the long-term, one is more likely to get diabetes. Further, the informer indicates that polycystic ovary syndrome (PCOS) affects women in different ways and it's hard to tell what will happen to them. It all depends on what symptoms one gets and whether one decides to have treatment or not. However, in the long-term, one is more likely to get diabetes. This may be because women with PCOS have trouble regulating the amount of sugar in their blood. This happens to between 1 and 10 in 100 women with PCOS. The chances increase if you are overweight.

In my case both the syndrome and the overweight issue were there. Since my menstrual periods started, I had experienced heavy bleeding during the menses and in 1996; I was diagnosed with a 4.6cm right ovarian cyst. However, I took no action except hygienic and proper personal care during the menses. In 1999, I went for a recheck and the cyst had increased to 5.6cm, still I continued as before. In 2002, I could not ignore the problem any longer and another check showed that the cyst was still there, this time with a slight reduction to 5.2cm. My Doctor recommended that it be surgically removed which was done. The difference between my cyst and the POCS is that mine was one huge cyst whereas POCS involves multiple small cysts but diseases don't read books so my guess is that in one way or the other, the condition might have predisposed me to diabetes.

On the issue of weight, my height is 1.57m and at the time of diabetes onset, I was 87kgs giving a body mass index (BMI) of 35.3(BMI which was calculated using the formula $BMI=kg/h^2$ where h is the height). A BMI of 30-40 falls in the obese category. According to Taylor[7] in the diabetes care, in any group of people with type 2 diabetes, simple inspection reveals that diabetes develops in some with a body mass index (BMI) in the normal or overweight range, whereas others have a very high BMI. In my case, the fact that my weight had an input in the development of diabetes is not questionable.

## 1.2.5 Other predisposing factors

Many other factors that contributed to my diabetic situation include age, limited exercise, stress, solitary life and overworking. I was over 50 years of age at the time of diagnosis and 5 years prior to this, I had changed my career from a field officer to an office staff. This means that I spent my whole day seated doing administrative work which was very stressing as compared to the field exercise. It also meant that I had minimal physical exercise. In addition to that, my children had grown up and left home and being a single mum meant that I spent most of my evenings with the house help. In-fact most of the evenings were spent on the computer trying to finalize office work. The office activities were also new to the routine professional work that I had carried out before and it meant reading a lot to update my skills on the same. At the office too it was not easy as the new job had its demands and relationships. This meant that I used to sleep not earlier than midnight and wake up by 6 am the following day. Further, I had disagreed with a close friend and some close family members on different issues and this caused a lot of stress. I also had an important activity that required consultation and having fallen out with my confidants, I had to solve the issue unaided. This was very stressful and I belief predisposed me to the condition.

## 1.2.6 Late symptoms of diabetes

In the week of the diagnosis, I had experienced weakness,  continuous tiredness likely to cause fainting, loss of appetite, plus numbness and tingling of the fingers and toes. The weakness and tiredness could be as a result of not eating the whole weak as I was only consuming processed orange and purple passion fruit juices. It could also be due to the fact that glucose was not being transported from the blood to the cells so as to generate energy as is the case of a non-diabetic person. The loss of appetite on the other hand could have been as a result of ketoacidosis. Diabetic ketoacidosis (DKA) is a complication that occurs when high levels of ketones build up in the blood and urine. According to University of Iowa Health Care[8], when your body does not produce enough insulin, the cells are unable to use glucose for fuel. As a result, the body begins breaking down fat for energy, a process, which produces ketones. Symptoms of diabetic ketoacidosis include loss of appetite, significant weight loss, frequent urination and confusion. Vomiting is another sign of ketoacidosis that requires immediate medical attention as loss of consciousness and coma may occur.

Over time, abnormally high blood sugar levels will cause damage to the body's nerves, a condition called diabetic neuropathy. While not all people experience this symptom, more advanced cases of diabetes may notice numbness, tingling, or pain in their extremities, typically starting with the feet. This symptom is most common in people who have had type 2 diabetes for 25 years or more, but it can occur in people who are in the early stages as well.

According to Mayo clinic[9] the cause of nerve symptoms isn't completely clear, but combinations of factors are likely to play a role, these include the complex interaction between nerves and blood vessels. High blood sugar interferes with the ability of the nerves to transmit signals. It also weakens the walls of the small blood vessels (capillaries) that supply the nerves with oxygen and nutrients. Depending on the affected nerves, symptoms of diabetic neuropathy can range from pain and numbness in the extremities (feet and hands) to problems with the digestive system, urinary tract, blood vessels and heart. For some people, these symptoms are mild; for others, diabetic neuropathy can be painful, disabling and even fatal. Diabetic neuropathy is a common serious complication of diabetes. Yet you can often prevent diabetic neuropathy or slow its progress with tight blood sugar control and a healthy lifestyle. In my case the condition was mild.

## 2. POST DIABETES DIAGNOSIS

Two years post diagnosis; I had controlled diabetes to an extent of not taking any medication at all. This was through a rigorous regime that used a combination of foods, exercise plus record keeping on important parameters that include blood pressure, body weight and glycemic index (GI). The post diagnosis period is divided into 5 stages. The first stage is between May and June 2014 post hospitalization and which involved intense medication that comprised of insulin injection among other medication. Stage 2 (July -December 2014) that involved non-injectable medication and close monitoring of foods, GI, blood pressure and weight. The third stage is between January and May 2015 when food took the center stage. The fourth stage is June - December 2015 when no medication was in use but the Glycemic index was above 6.0. The fifth and last stage is January to May 2016 when no medication was in use but the Glycemic index was below 6.0.


2.1: Stage 1(May -June 2014) - Intense Injectable and Non-Injectable Medication

This is between one and two months post diagnosis. At diagnosis, the GI was 30.8mml/l (normal is less than 6) and the $HBA_{1C}$ was 11.4 %( normal is approximately 5%). The provisional (unconfirmed) diagnosis was diabetes and hypertension and at discharge, the diagnosis (confirmed) was "newly diagnosed diabetes/hypertension". As soon as I was discharged, I procured a whole blood glucose meter and related accessories (Figure 2) and one month later a digital blood pressure monitor for the wrist (Figure 3). I also purchased a book on diabetes ''A Practical guide to health- Scientific and nutritional treatments) [10], a book on how to add years to your life and life to your years also known as " The little book of Health for seniors"[11], a book on Family nutrition, an FAO[12] publication and also a book on  applied basic Agri-nutrition[13] by the Kenya Ministry of Agriculture and Ministry of Public Health and Sanitation. Equipped with the tools and the literature, I set on the diabetes control journey.

**Glycemic Index (GI)**

The initial GI reading (5 days post discharge) was 11.5 and it was taken in the evening before meals and before any medication. Subsequent readings were taken first thing after waking up (fasting glycemia or fasting blood glucose) and the other one just before dinner. The readings were designed to be taken on all days but sometimes it was not possible due to work related timings. During the days that it was taken, the highest fasting blood glucose was 10.8 and the lowest 6.3. The average was 8.4. As for the evening glucose, the highest was 11.5 and the lowest 6.2 and the average was 7.4(Annex 1). The fasting plasma (blood) glucose was therefore above 7. The world health organization (WHO)[14] gives a sustained   greater or equal to fast blood glucose (GI) of 7 as the diagnostic criteria for diabetes and although this figure might not exactly tally with that from other health bodies such as the American Diabetic Association (ADA) as it was found out by Choi and others[15], it is an indication that my blood sugar remained high post discharge though far much less than the 30.8 at admission. However, there was a gradual decline in readings with time. The same continued into the following month and when the GI became consistently less than 8, the stringent taking of this parameter was reduced to once a day and this was the fasting reading in the morning.

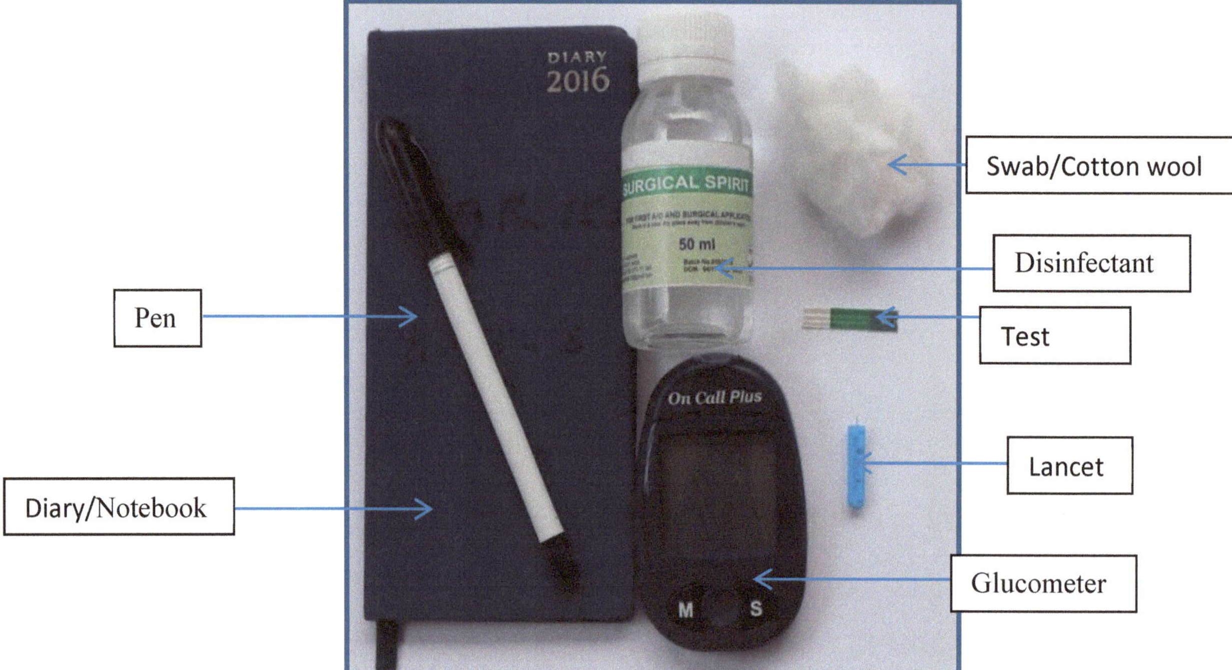


Figure 2: Blood glucose meter and related accessories

**Medication**

The medication that was issued out at discharge time from the hospital included that of diabetes (Insulin and Metformin), blood pressure and others. Soluble insulin was injected below the skin (subcutaneously) in the morning and evening just after the GI reading. The dose was at a gradual reducing level by 2 units for both the morning and evening doses. The start dose for the morning was 20 units and that of the evening was 10. The criterion used to reduce the dosage was the GI reading. A significant GI reduction was followed by a 2 unit insulin reduction in both occasions. In the first week of the second month, the zero dosage was reached and at that time, the GI was 7.2 and few days after it was 7 or thereabout. This encouraged total withdrawal of the insulin. During the same period the other medications continued especially the oral treatment of diabetes with metformin XR at the rate of 2 tablets of 500mgs in the morning only.

At this time, the relationship between the medication and the GI readings had not been taken as an important factor but as the taking of the readings continued, a number of issues raised some interest. It was noted that at the early stages of treatment that is the first month, forgetting to take metformin or inject insulin lead to a rise in the GI the following day, however as the days went on, withdrawal of insulin did not lead to rise of the GI and latter even forgetting to take metformin for one day did not have a very big effect on the GI level. This was the light at the end of the tunnel as it was an indication that at some time, the metformin might also be withdrawn just like insulin.

**Diet**

During the period under discussion, recording of the diet had not been given much consideration and a note was only recorded when there was a significant fluctuation of the GI reading the day after a certain meal was taken. Further, although it had been made clear at hospital discharge time that an overhaul in diet was important from the current high carbohydrate and fat to a low status of the same, the message had not sunk in and only a few changes like complete withdraw of sugar in tea and reducing the amount of food consumed per each of the 3 meals (breakfast, Lunch and dinner) had been made in as far as diet is concerned. However, as medication continued and record keeping was sustained, it was noted that taking a sugary meal before taking the GI reading led to a sharp rise in the GI. For example taking a glass of sweetened orange juice 2 hours before measurement of GI activated a rise in 2 units of the reading as compared to a similar analysis the previous day. Another factor that was noted was that eating some foods ended up with a significant reduction in the GI. Some of these foods include local chicken and arrow roots. The regularity of the meals also affected the GI reading in that when lunch was taken late and the mid-morning tea was taken with a snack, the GI levels went up. The above findings were another milestone that encouraged strict recording on the menus, in an attempt to identify the effect of each one of them on the GI. However, the findings might not be new scientifically in that an undisputable way of confirming if an individual has diabetes or not is through a test known as oral glucose tolerance test (OGTT) or oral glucose overload test (OGOT).This is a test that is done when the others have not been conclusive. According to World Health Organization (WHO) [14], diabetes is confirmed if the GI is greater or equal to 11.1 mmol/l, 2 hours (2-h) after taking a meal.


**Blood pressure**

While diabetes diagnosis came hand in hand with that of hypertension, the later has been given a cold shoulder or relegated to back stage in this book. This is because the only indication of hypertension that I had experienced so far was the short-lived increased heart beats once in a while before diagnosis of the same plus the high reading during the diagnosis time. Due to this thinking, the blood pressure medication was not continued with after the initial dose came to an end 14 days after discharge. This is not a physician's advice but personal decision. This assumption is not peculiar to me alone, the world Health Organization (WHO) [16] states that most hypertensive people have no symptoms at all and that there is a common misconception that people with hypertension always experience symptoms, but the reality is that most hypertensive people have no symptoms at all. Sometimes hypertension causes symptoms such as headache, shortness of breath, dizziness, chest pain, palpitations of the heart and nose bleeds. It can be dangerous to ignore such symptoms, but neither can they be relied upon to signify hypertension. Hypertension is a serious warning sign that significant lifestyle changes are required. The condition can be a silent killer and it is important for everybody to know their blood pressure reading

During the period under discussion, blood pressure was only taken 3 times with the first being immediately after purchase of the gadget. The first reading was 176/85/82. Where 176 is the systolic, 85 the diastolic and 82 the heartbeat. According to the world Health Organization (WHO) [16], blood pressure is measured in millimeters of mercury (mm Hg) and is recorded as two numbers, usually written one above the other. The upper number is the systolic blood pressure - the highest pressure in blood vessels and happens when the heart contracts, or beats. The lower number is the diastolic blood pressure -the lowest pressure in blood vessels in between heartbeats when the heart muscle relaxes. Normal adult blood pressure is defined as a systolic blood pressure of 120 mm Hg and a diastolic blood pressure of 80 mm Hg. However, the cardiovascular benefits of normal blood pressure extend to lower systolic (105 mm Hg) and lower diastolic blood pressure levels (60 mm Hg). Hypertension is defined as a systolic blood pressure equal to or above 140 mm Hg and/or diastolic blood pressure equal to or above 90 mm Hg. Normal levels of both systolic and diastolic blood pressure are particularly important for the efficient function of vital organs such as the heart, brain and kidneys and for overall health and wellbeing. According to the Centers for disease Control and Prevention (CDC) [17], the heartbeat of a 50 year old is between 85 and 119 beat per minute (bpm). From the first reading, it is obvious that the figures are well above the normal notwithstanding the fact that I was on hypertension reduction medication. However, I consoled myself with the fact that this was the first reading and inexperience or the excitement of using the tool for the first time might have contributed to the high reading

The second was taken the following day and the reading was 138/70/71 which is not too far from the recommended. The third pressure data was taken 12 days after the second reading and it was 126/70/77. This is a marked improvement either on data collection or the heart parameters being measured or both.

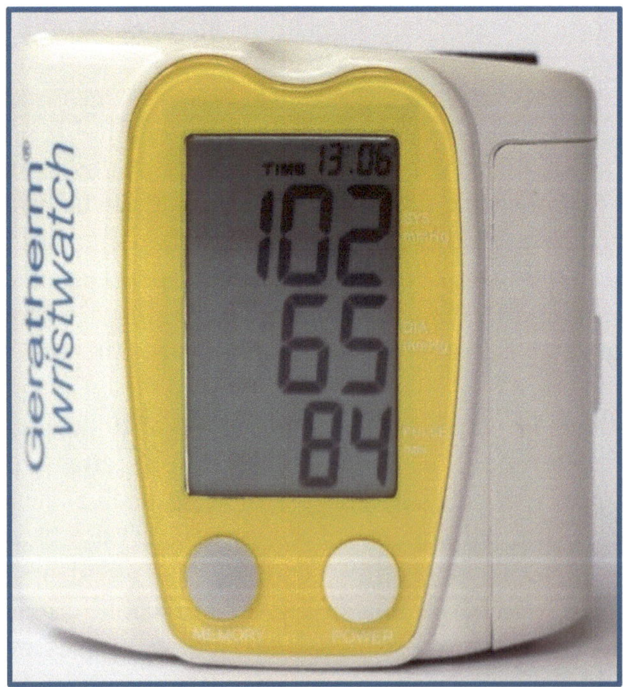


Figure 3: Digital blood pressure monitor for the wrist

**Glycemic Index (GI)**

Recording of the GI had now reduced to a few days in a month that is in the morning before medication. The decision to take a reading depended on availability of time which in turn depended on scheduled activities for the day in the office. It was also prompted by suspicion that the GI might be too high or too low depending on what was consumed the previous day especially dinner. During that period, the readings were between 5.9 and 8.4 (refer to Annex 2) and the average was 6.6. Only in 2 instances was the GI above 8 and similarly, only in 2 occasions did it fall below 6. This was a great improvement from the previous review period. During the two occasions that the GI was above 8, it was noted that the diets included either forgetting to take medication the previous day or taking too much carbohydrates the preceding day. Overeating too had the same effect on GI. The low readings below 5.9 were preceded by consuming a light meal for dinner such as fruit salad or just fruits. Foods that had been noted to have a low GI such as local Chicken and green peas were also found to have been part of the meals taken the day before a low GI reading. Other foods that were also found to be followed by a low GI included French beans, brown rice, pork, Fish and African night shade vegetables.

**Medication**

The medication in the initial part of this stage involved 2 tablets of Metformin XR taken once before breakfast. However, in the latter section of this stage(from November), it was noted that forgetting to take the medication did not have a very big change in the GI reading and taking one tablet in one of the days did not have a significant change in the GI too. One tablet of Metformin XR was thus adopted for medication from this point onwards. The other medication taken once during the period under review was calcium. This was necessitated by a feeling of weakness in the hip joint. Prior to diabetes diagnosis, I had a culture of taking calcium tablets whenever I felt weakness of the said joints especially when excessive pressure had been exerted on them either by a heavy load or over-walking. This used to be a quick and short term remedy that used to be discontinued as soon as the symptoms disappeared.

**Diet**

Food had already been identified as key to lowering the GI, however, strict recording of the consumed foods had not been adopted and this could have been one of the factors undermining attainment of the desired GI. Despite this setback, more and more foods that reduced the GI continued to be identified in all the categories of grains and tubers, animal and plant proteins, vegetables and fruits, fats, oils and nuts. Although this is not news as it is there in literature, it was confirmed that consuming white meat such as pork, local chicken and boiled fish had a significant reduction in the GI. Food preparation and composition of ingredients too had some effect on the GI an example being consuming mashed black beans versus one that is not mashed. The latter had a lower GI probably because the mash was composed of green maize, black beans, green bananas and Irish potatoes while the one that was not mashed was composed of green maize, black beans and vegetables. Thus a combination of the consumed foods was also being noted especially if it had significant effect on the GI. As mentioned in the Glycemic index section above, foods such as white meat, African night shade vegetables were followed by low GI records. Towards the end of the period under review, it was found out that consistent utilization of these foods    followed by a variation of the foods in the categories say taking local chicken one day, fish the day led to a consistently low GI. This encouraged consumption of such foods with amazing results.

**Blood pressure**

Blood pressure was taken irregularly during this period, and the only consideration that opted taking of the reading was time. This was so especially when the office and or personal schedules were not tight. This means that the blood pressure was taken during moments of relaxation. The highest set of readings was 137/80/87 which interprets to systolic pressure of 137, diastolic pressure of 80 and a heart (pulse) rate of 87. The lowest set on the other hand was 107/64/79. There was no significant relationship between the GI and the blood pressure at this time, nor was any relationship between the foods and blood pressure noted.

**Body Weight/Exercise**

As indicated earlier on, my weight pre-diagnosis was 87kgs and a body mass index was 35.3, placing me in the category of obese people. At discharge time, exercise and diet were highly recommended. I therefore, embarked on moderate and regular exercise which included most of the physical exercises I learnt during my primary school days. This includes running, walking, dancing, weight lifting and so on. Regularity here implies twice a week that is at the beginning of the week and mid-week. The duration was between 1 and 2 hours. These took place within the confines of my home compound. By December 2014, I was 72kgs which implies that I had lost 15kgs. These were the readings that were taken using the bathroom weighing scale that I had purchased (Figure 4). Prior to that, readings had been taken from public pay machines in the town center and records had just been memorized with no written record.

It has been noted before that *"Regular exercise is great for building muscle and losing fat, but if one want to see real weight-loss results, what one eat matters. But dropping pounds isn't about depriving oneself — it's about choosing the right foods that satisfy without the calories. Overhauling ones diet is an important place to begin if one wants to lose weight."*

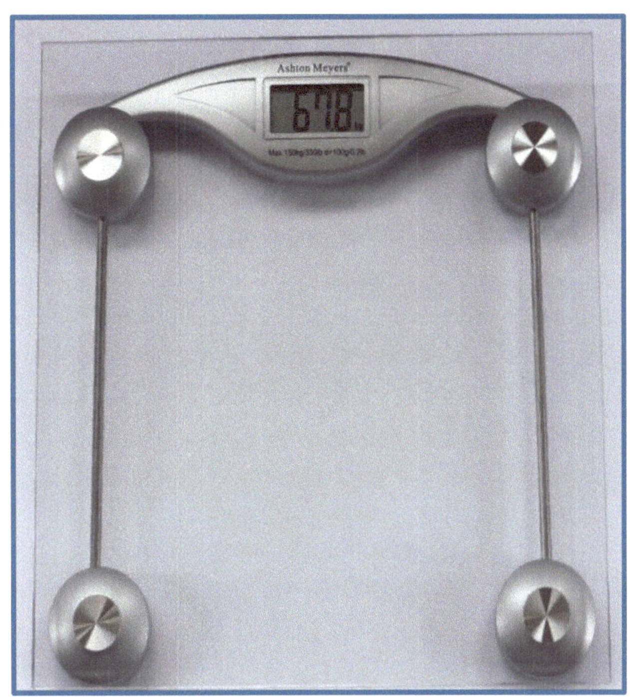

Figure 4: The bathroom weighing scale

2.3: Stage 3: January-May 2015: Diet takes Center stage

**Medication/GI and Blood Pressure**
This is nine to fourteen months post diagnosis and medication in the initial four months comprised of one tablet of Glucophage® (Metformin XR). The glycemic index (GI) varied between 6.1 and 7.7 with an average of 6.8. In the Month of May, Glucophage was withdrawn completely so as to assess how the body would cope without medication. During the withdrawal period, the GI fluctuated between 6.2 and 7.4 with an average score of 6.6. These readings compare favorably with those of the first four months when I was taking medication and it was concluded that the relatively low level of GI could be attributed to other management factors other than medication. This led to complete withdrawal of the drug. However, workload was high in the office and there was pulsation of the blood vessels adjacent to the ears. This was an indication of stress and high blood pressure and it necessitated consumption of a drug to reduce the same. Asomex®-5 which contains S (-) Amlodipine Besilate was used. In the last week of May, the pressure dropped from 132/75/79 to 105/74/70 and Asomex-5® was withdrawn.

**Diet**
Having discovered that consistent consumption of certain foods had significant effects in reducing GI, food at this stage took center stage with strict recording of what was consumed not only for dinner but for all the meals of the day that is breakfast, 10 & 4 o'clock snacks and lunch.

Breakfast consisted mostly of a fruit, an occasional protein, carbohydrate or some nuts or vegetables, all taken with a cup of tea (Annex 3). The fruits were chosen from a long list of locally available products depending on the season and that included bananas, mangoes, pawpaw, passion fruits, plums, melon, oranges, pineapple and white supote. The list of proteins included a portion of fish, sausage (beef/chicken/pork), milk, ovals (liver, kidney) eggs, beans and peas. It is important to note that milk was only taken with Weetabix and not plain as had been the case before. The amount had been reduced from a 200mls cup to a 50ml glass. This is after recognizing that milk contain a lot of carbohydrates with a likely effect of raising the GI. The carbohydrates were those with complex sugars such arrow roots and sweet potatoes. Other carbohydrates were chapatis which are made of wheat and; Weetabix also from wheat. It is important to note that prior to the diagnosis, the trend was to consume white bread with butter or margarine but in this case, the roots were boiled and the chapatis and Weetabix were made of whole wheat grains flour. This means that they had a lot of fiber. The idea here is to take carbohydrates that digest slowly thus releasing small amounts of glucose over a long period as opposed to highly digestible ones such as white bread that spikes blood glucose within a short time. In the latter case, the high glucose level is acted on by a limited amount of insulin that is being produced or that is active against the sugars and the situation leads to a rise in the GI. The nuts included groundnut, cashew nuts and almonds while the vegetables included Spinach, kunde (cowpea leaves) and vegetable salad made of combinations of tomatoes, carrots, onions, capsicum, Chinese parsley [Dania]).

Ten and four  O'clock snacks were mostly fruits that included potions of bananas, mangoes, pawpaw, passion fruits, plums, melon, oranges, pineapple white supote, apples and pears. Other snacks included plain yogurt, groundnuts and while attending workshops, the list could extend to tea, samosa, sausage, banana or crisps, pop corns and even chocolate.

Lunch was similar to breakfast in terms of the ingredients that is fruit, proteins carbohydrates and vegetables. However, the variety list for each group of foods was bigger with fruits' list including others such as avocado. The proteins' list was even bigger with added products such as chicken, pork, goat meat, beef, lentils, Turkey, green gram, butter beans and French beans. The carbohydrates were even more and they comprised of roast potatoes, brown Ugali (made of a mixture of millet, sorghum and cassava flours), pasta (macaroni), and brown rice, mashed food with a mixture of maize, beans or peas mashed together with Irish potatoes and green bananas or both, yams, maize and beans stew. The list of vegetables was even longer and it extended to African nightshade (managu), cabbage, kales (sukuma wiki), pumpkin and pumpkin leaves, Amaranthus (terere), summer squash (Courgettes) and eggplant (Mbiriganya). Nuts were absent or rarely taken during lunch while tea was replaced with just plain water, warm lemon water or hot water with apple cider vinegar and with honey (ACVH). The latter was only taken when I was at home. It is important to note that vegetables were given prevalence and were included in every meal unlike before diagnosis where they were rare or in low quantities. The aim of including the vegetables is because they are high in fiber thus lowering the late of metabolism and the rate at which food constituents especially glucose is absorbed. Another change that had been made is that of the common meal (Ugali). Before diagnosis, Ugali used to be made from sifted maize floor that had very low fiber. However, after diagnosis, Ugali was made from high fiber sorghum and millet plus a complex carbohydrate tuber (cassava). When Ugali from maize was desired, the one made from maize whose flour was not sifted was consumed. The principle is the same that is of decreasing metabolism rate.

Dinner resembled lunch in as far as the ingredients (fruits, proteins and carbohydrates) are concerned and also in the combination of the ingredients. Added fruits include thorny melon that is said to have very low sugars and hence good for those with diabetes (Figure 5). It is also said to be rich in vitamins A and E. Another inclusion is the white supote fruit (Figure 6), a very sugary fruit that appeared to have a low GI.  Plain Yogurt (without added sugars) was also taken once in a while, newly introduced vegetables included Cauliflower and Broccoli both of which are high in fiber and low in carbohydrates

The deviation of pre-diagnosis at this stage is that fruits that were half ripe were preferred to over ripe ones. This was assumed that they have lower amounts of sugars and for sure, the GI readings confirmed the same. Hot water with lemon/honey and apple cider vinegar were also taken more frequently. Both are acidic in nature and had been recommended by a nutritionist as substances that aid in lowering the glycemic index.

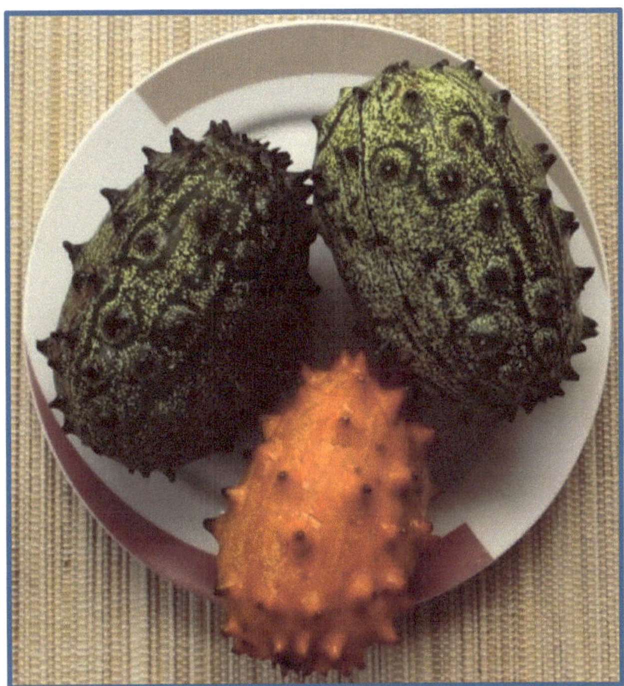

Figure 5: Thorny melon-Not ripe (T) and ripe (B)

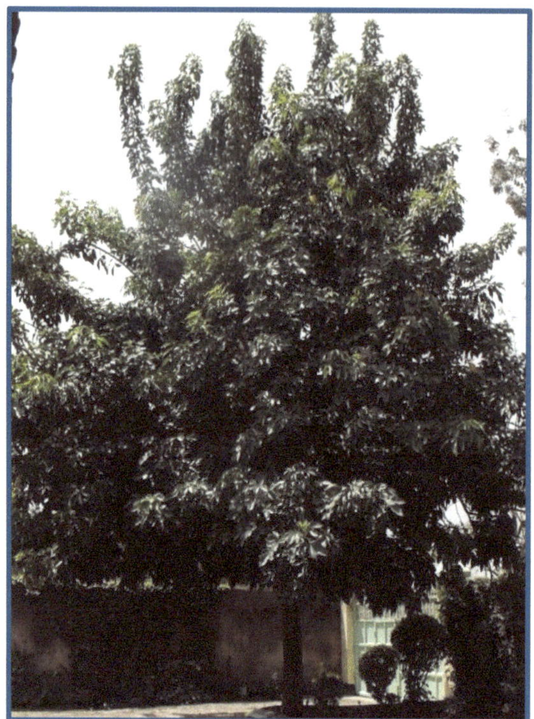 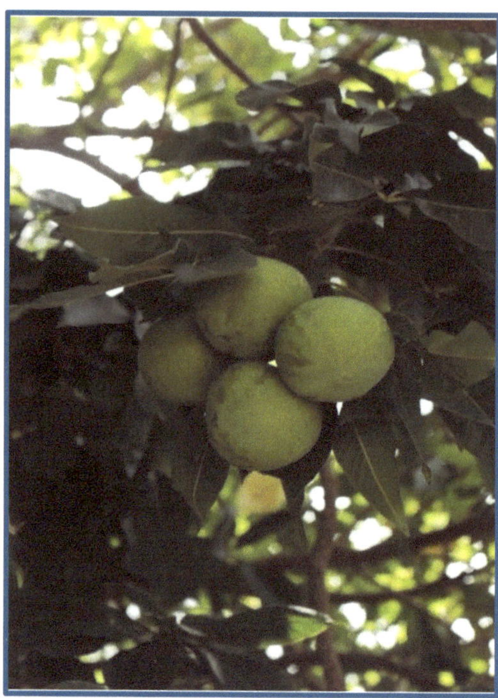

Figure 6: White Supote Tree (L) and Branch with Fruits (R)

## Body Weight/Exercise

The weight within this period was between 70.6 and 72kgs, an insignificant deviation from the previous stage. The reasons for the constant weight were not very clear but at least the weight was maintained at or below 72kgs.


2.4: Stage 4(June -December 2015)- No Diabetic medication , Glycemic Index above 6mmol/l
## Medication/GI and Blood Pressure
This is fourteen to 20 months post-diagnosis. The average GI was 6.5 and the range was between 6 and 7.7.  Pressure fluctuated between 143/89/74 and 103/66/77. The controlling factor for the pressure was at one time assumed to be Asomex-5® as when the pulsation of the head blood vessels next to the ears would be so high the drug would be consumed, however, it was noted that even at times when the pressure was as low as 106/59/68, the pulsations were still there. This necessitated a visit to a doctor who recommended a painkiller by the name pynstop® (Acetaminophen). In his opinion, the pulsation was due to headache as a result of stress. It somehow worked and was only used when there was a headache or pulsation.
 At this stage, it is very clear that the author had a phobia for hospitals and stuck to self-medication in most cases as opposed to medical prescriptions. This is not a peculiar phenomena to the writer. A study carried out "Wakenya report" during the compilation of this work showed that, although personal health ranks first among Kenyans as compared to personal comfort and family, 42% of Kenyans prefer self-medication or homemade remedies over seeing a doctor. The

41% who go to hospital are those in the higher earning status, perhaps because of the expensive health care[18]. In my opinion, other factors that discourage medical consultations include the age difference of the patient and the medic especially when the physician is younger and more so of the opposite sex. The reception that is accorded the patient by the doctor also matters; for example if the patients if welcomed in a manner that shows that s/he is too old say like "welcome old mama/woman", one feels too old to need medical services. Other restricting services include the perceived qualification and or experience of the medic, for example if you visit a hospital and you expect to meet a qualified medical doctor, and the one you find has no tag to confirm the same, then there is loss of confidence in the person. These are just a few and the list is endless.

**Diet/ Body weight/Exercise**

The meals remained more or less what was there in stage 3 and the physical activities remained the same with corresponding relative stage 3 weight of between 71.1 and 72.2

2.5 Stage 5(January to May 2016): No medication – GI less than 6mmol/l

**Glycemic Index/ Blood pressure/ Medication**
This is the period 21 to 25 months post diagnosis that is roughly two years. During this period, the GI was between 4.7 and 6.4. The average was 5.6 and out of the 38 GI readings that were taken, only 4 translating to 10% was above 6. In the month of January, laboratory results (Table 1) showed that the Glycosylated hemoglobin (HbA1c)) was 6.5%. This was a great improvement from the 11.4% in April 2014. The figure 6 was important in that the reference book that I was using[5] indicate that the fasting GI for a diabetic person should be between 4.5 and 6 while less than 7.8 can still be acceptable. In the case of a non-diabetic person, GI should be less than 5.6. The reference material also showed that the HbA1c for a diabetic should be less than 6.5% while less than 7.5% can still be acceptable. For a non-diabetic person, the HbA1c should be less than 6%. The laboratory results therefore showed that I was starting to control diabetes as the GI average reading of 5.6 was within the desired 4.5 to 6 for a diabetic person.
The lowest pressure record during this period was 120/64/56 while the highest was 150/78/72. The latter which is one of the two times during this period that the systolic pressure was above 135 was associated with attainment of a GI of less than 6, something that I had been striving to achieve. The high pressure was therefore was not given any medical attention. Other parameters such as blood cholesterol were also showing favorable signs of control except Triglycerides that I needed to work on (Table 1).
 During this period, no diabetes or high blood pressure medication was taken. However, a prescription of atorvastatin 10mg was prescribed to reduce triglycerides to the desired 1.71 mmol/L from 3.65 mmol/L obtained during the laboratory test.

Table 1: Laboratory results of blood analysis in January 2016

| TEST | RESULTS | UNITS | DESIRABLE | STATUS |
|---|---|---|---|---|
| Total cholesterol | 4.93 | Mmol/l | <5.2 | N |
| HDL | 1.74 | Mmol/l | >1.41 | N |
| Triglycerides | 3.65 | Mmol/l | <1.71 | H |
| LDL | 1.52 | Mmol/l | <3.6 | N |
| TC/HDL | 2,8 |  | <4 | N |
| HbA1c | 7.2 | % | <6.5 | H |

Note:
- The urinalysis results also indicated the absence of glucose, proteins, ketones, Nitrites, bilirubin and urobilinogen in urine and the pH was 7.0.This was a big improvement from that of +2 for glucose and blood as at the diagnosis time in April 2014
- Exceptional Figures are highlighted in Yellow

**Diet/ Body weight/Exercise**

The body weight fluctuated between 67.3 and 72 with an average of 69.3. On the 35 times that the weight readings were taken, only 6(17%) of the cases was above 70kgs. This was a great improvement from the previous stage where the weight was always above 70kgs. The lowest weight of 67.3kgs shows a monumental reduction of 19.7 kgs from that of 87 kgs at diagnosis.

The progressive data analysis in this investigation shows that there is a correlation between the weight and the GI as both appear to decline with time. The bridging factor in both of them is the diet. In this stage, the food groups remained more or less the same as what was consumed in stage 4, however in this stage, a few changes were made that are believed to have led to the reduced weight and blood sugars. One key change that was made was to reduce the potions of other food groups (carbohydrates, proteins, fruits etc.) and increase the ratio of the vegetables. This assisted in reducing the amount of food consumed without feeling hungry in-between the meals mainly because of the high fiber content of the vegetables. Another change that always indicated a drastic reduction of blood sugars the following morning is replacement of the normal diet with a fruit salad in plain yoghurt the previous night. This discovery has not only assisted in maintaining a low blood sugar but has also made it possible to maintain weight which as I write this article in July 2017 is between 66 and 67kgs. The significant results noted when minimal amounts of consumables were taken during dinner time confirmed the saying that states *"Eat breakfast like a king, lunch like a prince, and dinner like a pauper"*. The fact that the diet was considered as the most important activity that controlled the weight, blood sugars and blood pressure affirmed another adage that says *"Eat food like medicine or else you will eat medicine like food"*. As for fruits, it was noted that consuming half ripe ones such as mangoes led to a low GI. Further, consuming them with their outer-cover (peels) reduced the GI even further. In conclusion, the role played by diet in control of diabetes cannot be understated.

### 3. LESSONS LEARNT

1. It is good to take a rest from work for a while so as to stabilize the blood sugars
2. Regularity of meals is very important. Strictly adhere to meal times as variation in timing one day's meal can raised the GI significantly the following day
3. Quantities consumed especially if they are high in carbohydrates and fats affect the GI. The higher the quantities, the higher the GI.
4. Steady decrease of the consumed quantities of the meals of the day (breakfast, lunch and Dinner) leads to lower levels of GI the following day and the meals are also able to supply adequate energies when they are required most. Thus *"Eat breakfast like a king, lunch like a prince, and dinner like a pauper"*.
5. Replacing beef with goat meat lowers the GI. This could be due to the fact beef has a higher level of fat than goat meat (32% of the recommended daily intake of fat in 100 grams of beef as opposed to 5% in goat meat of the same weight) [13]. This could be due to the fact that fats are next in line in provision of energy after carbohydrates.
6. Some sugary foods might lower the GI instead of raising it. These include carrots, sweet potatoes and green peas. Literature[13] confirms that they are very low in carbohydrates and fat (2 and 0 for green peas and 6 and 0 for sweet potatoes respectively). Their sweetness could be from sugars other than glucose. For example sweet potatoes have a mixture of sucrose, glucose and fructose sugars in which case fructose is higher amounts than the other two combined.
7. Some high carbohydrate foods do not raise the GI as expected especially if they are consumed in moderate amounts. These include Irish potatoes, arrow roots and cassava. This could be due to the complex nature of the carbohydrates that takes time to break down to glucose thus releasing small amounts of sugar into the blood stream.
8. Nuts that include Almonds, Groundnuts, Cashew and walnuts might have glycemic reducing factors
9. The cooking method affects the GI. Deep fried foods- chicken, fish raised the GI despite being white meat while the boiled version of the same foods leads to low GI.
10. Soul search and scientific reasoning can provide the good will required to start taking the right diet. The extra 20 kgs that I lost are equivalent to carrying 20 lts water can with me everywhere I go. Shedding it makes my daily burden easier to carry( Figure 7)
11. Half ripe sugary fruits such as mangoes have lower GI than fully ripe ones. Further, consuming them with their cover peels lowers the GI even more.
12. Apart from diet, exercise and medication where necessary, if possible, one needs to invest in a few tools that aid the management of the disease. These include a glucometer and its accessories, a pressure gauge, a weighing scale or a simple tape measure to measure you waist regularly, a watch or clock preferably with set alarms to alert you when it is time to take a meal, some exercise materials like a simple rope, a track suit and so on
13. Diabetes is not a crime, it is important that you those stay with know that you have it. This way, they will understand when they see you taking a snack at the wrong time and or place. New fitting clothes as you continue to loose wait improves your confidence.
14. Regular medical checkup cannot be replaced by any literature, written or otherwise.

15. Early diagnosis and management of diabetes are key to prevention of advanced signs such as blindness.

16. Practice appropriate exercise; while in a story building walk up and down the stair, when in an open ground run a little bit, when in a closed community hit the gym, when in a limited space use the rope and skip and or dance etc

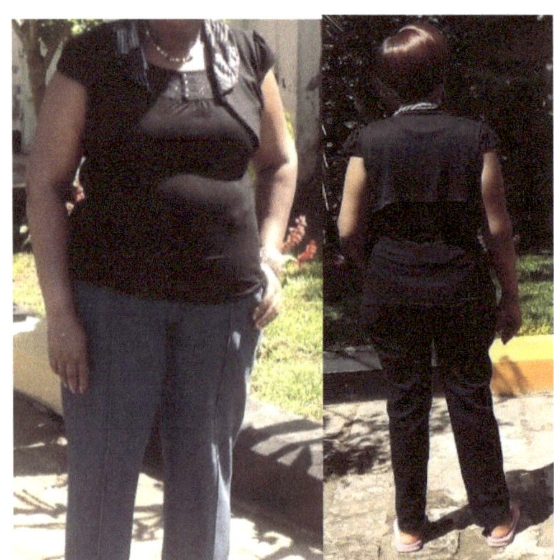

Figure 7: Author-Before diagnosis (L) and 2 years post diagnosis

# 4. ANNEXES



## Annex 1: Data on Stage 1(May 2014-June 2014) - Intense Injectable and Non-Injectable Medication

**May, 2014**

| Date | Glycemic Index(GI) (mml/l) -morning | Glycemic Index(GI) (mml/l) -evening | Insulin - Mixtard (units)- morning | Insulin - Mixtard (units)- evening | Blood Pressure (mmHg) | Oral Diabetes Medicine | Other Medicine | Remarks |
|---|---|---|---|---|---|---|---|---|
| 1-4 | - | - | 20 | 10 | - | Metformin 2x500mgs XR tabs– morning only, Diamicron- mr 60 at Night | Evening for all drugs, Aztor- I tab<br><br>Amlodipine- 5mg,<br><br>Neurofort-1 tab daily<br><br>Losatrim-<br><br>Tefloxycin- 500mgs- 1 week | Not yet purchased the glucometer and Pressure gauge |
| 5 | - | 11.5 | 20 | 10 | - | Metformin 2x500mgs XR tabs– morning only, Diamicron- mr 60 at Night | Amlodipine- 5mg,<br><br>Neurofort-<br><br>Aztor | Dinner at 9pm. Blood glucose reading before insulin injection |
| 6 | - | 11.1 | 20 | 10 | - | " | " | - |
| 7 | 10.8 | 7.3 | 18 | 8 | - | " | " | - |
| 8 | - | 7.4 | 18 | 18 | - | Metformin 2x500mgs XR tabs– morning only, | " | Mix up time for evening dose of insulin |
| 9 | 7.9 | 7.2 | 16 | 8 | - | - | " | Forgot to take Metformin |
| 10 | - | 9.2 | 14 | 6 | - | Metformin 2x500mgs XR tabs– morning only | " | - |
| 11 | 8.9 | 8.4 | 14 | 14 | - | " | " | - |
| 12 | 8.4 | 8.0 | 12 | 6 | - | " | " | - |
| 13 | 8.3 | 8.1 | 12 | 6 | - | " | " | - |
| 14 | 8.2 | 10.1 | 10 | 6 | - | " | " | Took a glass of Orange Fruit juice 2 hours before evening blood glucose reading |
| 15 | 8.6 | 6.8 | 10 | 6 | - | " | - | - |
| 16 | 8.1 | - | 10 | 6 | - | " | - | - |
| 17 | 7.0 | 6.2 | 8 | 4 | - | " | - | - |
| 18 | 6.3 | 5.7 | 8 | 4 | - | " | - | - |
| 19 | 6.3 | 6.2 | 6 | 4 | - | " | - | - |
| 20 | 7.5 | - | 4 | 4 | - | " | - | - |
| 21 | - | 9.3 | 4 | 4 | - | " | - | **Lunch:** Arrow Roots, Beef Sausage, Samosa at both **11 o'clock** **SNACK:** Same as lunch |
| 22 | - | 6.4 | 4 | 4 | - | " | - | - |
| 23 | 7.2 | 6.4 | 4 | 2 | - | " | - | Forgot morning Metformin |
| 24 | - | 6.2 | 4 | 2 | - | " | - | - |
| 25 | - | - | 4 | 2 | - | " | - | - |
| 26 | 8.4 | - | 4 | 2 | - | " | - | - |
| 27 | 7.4 | - | 4 | 2 | - | " | - | - |

| 28 | 7.1 | - | 4 | 2 | - | '' | - | Ate Arrow Roots, Sweet Potatoes |
| 29 | 9.3 | - | 0 | 4 | - | '' | - | Forgot morning insulin, doubled evening dose |
| 30 | 8.6 | - | 4 | 1 | - | '' | - | |
| 31 | - | - | 4 | 2 | - | '' | - | Forgot to take morning Metformin |



| Date | Glycemic Index(GI) (mml/l) -morning | Glycemic Index(GI) (mml/l) -evening | Insulin-Mixtard (units)- morning | Insulin - Mixtard (units)- evening | Blood Pressure (mmHg) | Oral Diabetes Medicine | Other Medicine | Remarks |
|---|---|---|---|---|---|---|---|---|
| 1 | 7.4 | - | 4 | 2 | - | Metformin 2x500mgs XR tabs– morning only | - | - |
| 2 | 6.9 | - | 2 | - | - | '' | - | - |
| 3 | - | - | - | 2 | - | '' | - | - |
| 4 | 7.2 | - | 2 | - | - | '' | - | - |
| 5 | 6.8 | - | 2 | - | - | '' | - | - |
| 6 | 7.2 | - | 2 | - | - | '' | - | - |
| 7 | 6.9 | - | - | - | - | Metformin 2x500mgs XR -tabs – morning only | - | Ate a lot of Chicken, Fish, Bananas |
| 8 | 7.7 | - | - | - | - | '' | - | - |
| 9 | 7.3 | - | - | - | - | '' | - | - |
| 10 | - | - | - | - | - | '' | - | - |
| 11 | - | - | - | - | - | '' | - | - |
| 12 | - | - | - | - | - | '' | - | - |
| 13 | 6.8 | - | - | - | 176/85/82 | '' | - | Excited at owning a Pressure gauge- 1st time to take own readings |
| 14 | 6.8 | - | - | - | 138/70/71 | '' | - | Recommended reading as per machine in use 120/80/80 or below |
| 15 | 6.9 | - | - | - | - | '' | - | - |
| 16 | 7.3 | - | - | - | - | '' | - | - |
| 17 | 7.4 | - | - | - | - | '' | - | - |
| 18 | - | - | - | - | - | '' | - | - |
| 19 | 7.6 | - | - | - | - | '' | - | - |
| 20 | - | - | - | - | - | '' | - | - |
| 21 | - | - | - | - | - | '' | - | - |
| 22 | - | - | - | - | - | '' | - | - |
| 23 | - | - | - | - | - | '' | - | - |
| 24 | - | - | - | - | - | '' | - | - |
| 25 | 6.8 | - | - | - | 126/70/77 | '' | - | - |
| 27 | 6.8 | - | - | - | - | Metformin 500mgx2 morning only | - | Changed Metformin XR to just Metformin --but still 500gms Xr tablet is coated and thus long acting |
| 28 | 7.2 | - | - | - | - | '' | - | - |
| 29 | 7.3 | - | - | - | - | '' | - | - |

Note: Exceptional figures highlighted in yellow

# Annex 2: Data on Stage 2(July -December 2014): Non-injectable medication



| Date | Glycemic Index(GI)- morning | Blood Pressure | Body weight (kgs) | Diabetes Medicine | Other Medicine | Remarks |
|---|---|---|---|---|---|---|
| 4 | - | 117/65/75 | - | Metformin | - | - |
| 6 | - | - | - | - | - | Forgot to take Metformin |
| 7 | 8.4 | - | - | Metformin | - | - |
| 13 | 6.6 | 126/74/72 | - | '' | - | - |
| 19 | - | - | - | '' | - | **Dinner : Black Beans Mash** |
| 20 | 7.8 | - | - | '' | - | - |
| 22 | - | - | - | '' | - | **Dinner : Black Beans Mash** |

| 23 | 7.7 | - | - | " | - | |
| 24 | 6.2 | - | - | " | - | **Dinner** : Rice, Beef/Kales stew |
| 26 | - | 123/71/75 | - | " | - | **Dinner** : white Ugali for lunch & Carrots |
| 27 | 8.2 | - | - | " | - | - |
| 30 | 6.8 | - | - | " | - | - |

**August,2014**

| Date | Glycemic Index(GI)-morning | Blood Pressure | Body weight (kgs) | Diabetes Medicine | Other Medicine | Remarks |
|---|---|---|---|---|---|---|
| 3 | 5.9 | - | - | Metformin | - | **6 o'clock SNACK:** Chicken, Peas stew, white Rice for **Dinner:** Black berries |
| 4 | - | 123/71/71 | - | " | - | - |
| 7 | 6.8 | - | - | - | - | - |
| 11 | 6.5 | - | - | - | - | Forgot to take Metformin, ate Green Grams stew, Rice |
| 13 | 7.8 | 133/80/87 | - | - | - | Not taken Metformin for 3 days |
| 16 | 6.2 | - | - | Metformin | - | **Lunch**: Kales, Peas<br>**Dinner** :  Ugali, African nightshade ,Lugwarts |
| 17 | 6.2 | - | - | " | - | **Dinner** : Fish and Rice |
| 18 | 7.5 | - | - | " | - | Overate the previous Night |
| 20 | 6.4 | 131/73/71 | - | " | - | **Dinner** : Pigeon Peas and Cabbage |
| 24 | 6.5 | 114/65/70 | - | " | 1 Calcium (Z-Cal$^R$)tablet | Weakness of joints especially hip joint |
| 26 | 6.8 | - | - | " | - | - |
| 30 | 6.8 | - | - | " | - | - |

**September,2014**

| Date | Glycemic Index(GI)-morning (mmol/l) | Blood Pressure | Body weight (kgs) | Diabetes Medicine | Other Medicine | Remarks |
|---|---|---|---|---|---|---|
| 3 | 7.2 | 124/79/74 | - | Metformin XR | - | Changed to Metformin XR |
| 5 | 6.4 | 123/75/70 | - | " | - | |
| 13 | 6.5 | | - | " | - | |
| 17 | 6.7 | - | - | - | - | Forgot Metformin, attended a funeral,  ate Maize/Beans/Greens Mash |
| 19 | - | 124/74/76 | 74.7 | Metformin XR | - | - |
| 21 | 6.8 | - | - | " | - | - |
| 29 | - | 122/75/76 | - | " | - | - |

**October, 2014**

| Date | Glycemic Index(GI)-morning | Blood Pressure | Body weight (kgs) | Diabetes Medicine | Other Medicine | Remarks |
|---|---|---|---|---|---|---|
| 1 | 8.2 | - | - | Metformin XR | - | **4pm  SNACK:** Roasted Maize and 2 Sweet Bananas |
| 5 | 6.7 | - | - | " | - | - |
| 15 | 7.7 | - | - | - | - | Forgot Metformin |
| 18 | 7.7 | - | - | Metformin XR | - | - |
| 20 | - | 127/75/79 | 75.2 | " | | - |
| 24 | 7.3 | - | - | " | - | - |
| 31 | 6.9 | - | - | " | - | **Dinner:** Carrots salad with roasted Irish Potatoes |

**November, 2014**

| Date | Glycemic Index(GI)-morning | Blood Pressure | Body weight (kgs) | Diabetes Medicine | Other Medicine | Remarks |
|---|---|---|---|---|---|---|
| 3 | 7.8 | - | - | Metformin | - | **Started exercise-Dancing**<br>**Dinner:** Black Beans |
| 4 | 6.7 | - | - | " | - | **Dinner:** Broccoli |
| 7 | 6.8 | 121/69/76 | - | " | - | **Dinner:** Black Beans<br><br>Passion Fruit |
| 8 | 7.8 | - | - | - | - | Forgot Metformin Yesterday |
| 10 | 7.3 | - | - | - | - | **Dinner:** Black Beans<br><br>Fruit Salad |

| 11 | 6.7 | 131/76/73 | - | Metformin | - | Forgot to record diet |
|---|---|---|---|---|---|---|
| 12 | 7.3 | - | - | 1X500mg Metformin XR | - | |
| 13 | 6.7 | - | - | Metformin | - | Fish<br>African  Night shade ,<br>Orange Fruit & Passion |
| 14 | 7.6 | - | - | '' | - | **Breakfast:** Tea ,Egg, Samosa<br>Spinach, White Bread,  Lemon<br>Two Slices Of Bread |
| 15 | 6.4 | - | - | '' | - | **Dinner:** Cabbage<br>Sweet Potato,<br>Passion Fruit, Tangerine |
| 16 | 6.6 | - | - | '' | - | **Dinner:** Mash( Peas, Maize, Irish Potatoes & Green Bananas),<br>Cabbage, Passion Fruit,<br>Tangerine |
| 17 | 6.5 | - | - | '' | - | **Dinner:** Fish/Ugali<br>African nightshade,<br>Tangerine Fruit |
| 23 | 6.8 | - | - | '' | - | **Lunch:** Chicken /Ugali<br><br>**Dinner:** Ugali /Cauliflower, |
| 29 | 6.4 | - | - | '' | - | Rice,  Passion, Pawpaw |

December, 2014

| Date | Glycemic Index(GI)-morning | Blood Pressure | Body weight (kgs) | Diabetes Medicine | Other Medicine | Remarks |
|---|---|---|---|---|---|---|
| 6 | 6.6 | - | - | Metformin | - | **Dinner:** Ugali,  Fish ,African nightshade |
| 7 | 7.3 | 121/72/72 | - | - | - | **Lunch:** French Flies<br><br>**Dinner:** Mashed food |
| 9 | - | - | 72 | - | - | **Dinner:** Black Beans Mukimo(Mashed Black Beans , Green Maize, Irish Potatoes and Green Bananas)<br><br>-Thorny Melon |
| 16 | 6.3 | - | - | - | - | - |
| 21 | - | 107/64/79 | - | Metformin | - | On leave |
| 23 | 7.6 | - | - | - | - | Not taken Metformin for 2 days |
| 24 | 6.9 | - | - | Metformin | - | **Dinner:** Maize and Beans, Carrots, Cabbages, Beef Stew |
| 28 | 7.1 | 116/76/71 | - | '' | - | **Breakfast:** white bread without vegetables<br>**Dinner:** Fruit salad |
| 29 | 5.9 | - | - | '' | - | **Dinner:** Green Peas, Pawpaw and sugarless(plain) yogurt |
| 30 | 6.5 | - | - | '' | - | **Dinner:** Fish, Black Beans, Kales |
| 31 | 6.1 | - | - | '' | ' | Dinner: Brown Rice, French Beans, Thorny Melon, half ripe Mango |

Note: Exceptional figures highlighted in yellow

# Annex 3: Data on Stage 3(January-May 2015: Diet takes Center stage

January, 2015

| Date | GI | Pressure | Wt. (kgs) | Breakfast | Snack 10am | Lunch | Snack 4pm | Dinner | Diabetes Medicine |
|---|---|---|---|---|---|---|---|---|---|
| 1 | 6.2 | - | - | - | - | - | Sweet Cake, Unripe Mango | Spaghetti, Cabbage/ Butter Nut Stew, Pawpaw, Thorny Melon in plain Yogurt, | Glucophage XR -1 Tablet |
| 2 | 6.7 | - | 72 | - | - | Chicken, Roast Potatoes, Cake | - | Green Peas stew, Brown Chapati, Pawpaw, | '' |

| | | | | | | | | | |
| --- | --- | --- | --- | --- | --- | --- | --- | --- | --- |
| | | | | | | | | Lemon/honey/ hot water | |
| 3 | 6.4 | 120/65/75 | - | Chapati, Fish | Mango | Green Peas stew, Chapati | - | Ugali , Offals/ African nightshade vegetables, Yogurt/ Thorny Melon | '' |
| 4 | 6.4 | - | - | Sweet Potatoes, Banana, Egg | Banana | Offals /African nightshade vegetables, Ugali | - | Mash Potatoes , Offals/ Cabbage/ Green Banana stew, Thorny Melon, Mango, Lemon /Honey tea | '' |
| 5 | 6.4 | | | Sweet Potato, Banana | Banana | Cabbage, Potato, Chapati | | Black Bean Mash, fried Beef/Carrots Salad , Lemon/ Honey tea | '' |
| 6 | 6.1 | - | - | Chapati, Sweet Potato, Banana, Tea | - | Cabbage, Rice, Spaghetti. | | Pork, Ugali Unga (flour) No. 2, Kales/Spinach . Melon, Lemon /Honey tea | '' |
| 7 | 6.4 | - | - | Weetabix/ Milk, Banana, Groundnuts | - | White Ugali ,Pork, Peas, Kales/Spin ach, 2 Mangoes | - | Rice, Beef/Pumpkin / Cabbage stew, 'Melon, Lemon/honey tea | '' |
| 8 | 6.6 | 135/76/76 | | Banana, Cashew nuts, Peanuts | - | Beef /Pumpkin/ Cabbage stew, Pork, Brown Rice, Sweet Banana | - | Chicken, Peas, Sukuma, Spinach, Potato Stew , White Flour Chapati | No Glucophage, Bread, Salad, |
| 9 | 6.4 | - | - | Bread, Butter, Mango, Peanuts, Cashew nuts | - | - | - | | '' |
| 10 | 6.9 | 130/76/65 | | Weetabix, milk, Banana, Pawpaw and Cashew nuts | Mango | Peas, meat, sandwich, Banana, milk shake and honey | sugarca ne | Peas, Rice, fruit salad, yogurt, honey and Lemon tea. | Glucophage, |
| 11 | 7.3 | 134/79/79 | - | Bread, butter, Pawpaw , Banana | - | Rice, Sukuma, Beef, fruit salad, yogurt | - | Mukimo, Black Beans, Cauliflower/ Broccoli/ Meat stew, Mango, Lemon / honey tea | - |
| 17 | 7.3 | - | - | Arrow Roots, Passion fruit, white bread, pea /Cashew nuts | Mango,- Peanuts | Mandazi, Samosa, Yam, Tea | - | Sweet Potatoes, Kamande(Len tils), Honey/Banan a | Glucophage |
| 18 | 6.5 | - | - | Bread/Vegeta ble salad, Sweet Banana | - | Amaranthu s, Bread, Chicken, Red Melon | - | Milkshake, Omena/Kunde , Ugali, Pawpaw, Lemon and | Glucophage |

| Date | GI | Pressure | Wt. (Kgs) | B/Fast | Snack 10am | Lunch | Snack 4pm | Dinner | Diabetes Medicine |
|---|---|---|---|---|---|---|---|---|---|
| | | | | | | | | honey tea | |
| 21 | 6.9 | 135/83/76 | - | Cupcake, Arrow Roots, Pumpkin | Plums | Rice, Cabbage/Pepper, 2 biscuits | - | Pork, Njahi(Black Beans), Avocado, Melon, Pepper, Apple cider and honey tea | Glucophage |
| 25 | 6.1 | - | - | Omena(lake Victoria Sardine Fish), White bread Vegetable salad, Mango, Banana | plain yogurt, Pawpaw | Peas, Rice | - | Cabbage, Rice | Glucophage |
| 31 | 6.3 | - | - | Cattle Kidney, Sweet Potato Pawpaw | bread, Sausage, Samosa | Mango juice, Groundnuts | - | Ugali, Kales, Beef/Lentils stew | Glucophage |

**February 2015**

| Date | GI | Pressure | Wt. (Kgs) | B/Fast | Snack 10am | Lunch | Snack 4pm | Dinner | Diabetes Medicine |
|---|---|---|---|---|---|---|---|---|---|
| 7 | 6.7 | - | - | Chapati, Plums , Peanuts | 3 Plums | Chicken, Peas, Chapati | 3 Plums | Meat, Cabbage, Rice Pawpaw, Plums, ACVH | Glucophage XR 500 mgx2 Morning |
| 14 | 6.8 | - | - | Margarine Bread , Banana | 3 Plums | White Rice, Chicken, Cabbage, Red Melon | 3 Plums | Roast Irish Potatoes, Fried Mutton, Carrots/ Onion Salad, Pawpaw | ' ' |
| 15 | 6.6 | - | - | Sweet Potatoes, Omena, Peanuts, Pawpaw | 3 Plums | Roasted Irish Potatoes, Fish-Nile Perch, Carrots/ Onion Salad, Plums ACVH | 3 Plums | Cabbage, Pumpkin, Chapati, Pawpaw ACVH | ' ' |
| 22 | 6.4 | - | | Sweet Potatoes, Nile Perch, Mango | 3 Plums | Local Chicken, Ugali, Sweet Bananas | 3 Plums | Peas Mukimo, Peas, Pawpaw, ACVH | ' ' |
| 28 | 6.3 | - | 70.6 | Sweet Potatoes Fish-Nile Perch, 2 Sweet Bananas, 2 Plums | 4 Plums | Brown Rice, Lentil/ Beef stew, Spinach | 2 Plums | Sweet Potatoes, Cabbage/ Beef stew, Red Melon, ACVH | ' ' |

**March, 2015**

| Date | GI | Pressure | Wt. (kgs) | B/Fast | Snack 10am | Lunch | Snack 4pm | Dinner | Diabetes Medicine |
|---|---|---|---|---|---|---|---|---|---|
| 14 | 6.1 | - | - | Arrow Root, Mango | Ndazi, Lemon | Rice, Peas/ Beef stew | 2 Sweet Bananas | Cabbage/ Beef stew, Sweet Potatoes, Thorny Melon, Lemon | ' ' |

| Date | GI | Pressure | Wt. (Kgs) | Breakfast | Snack 10am | Lunch | Snack 4pm | Dinner | Diabetes Medicine | |
|---|---|---|---|---|---|---|---|---|---|---|
| | | | | | | | | tea/honey | | |
| 15 | 6.4 | - | - | Sweet Potato, Fish-Nile Perch, Sweet Banana-White Supote fruit | - | Cabbage/Spinach/Beef stew, Rice | | Black Bean-Mukimo, Avocado, Thorny, AVCH | '' | |
| 21 | 7.3 | - | - | Spinach, Sausage, Porridge, Sweet Potatoes, Arrow root, Fruit salad (Banana, Melon, Orange Fruit) | Tea, Ndazi | Chicken, Beef, White Rice, White Chapati, Cabbage | Hot Lemon water, Ndazi | Ugali, Matumbo/Cauliflower Stew, Lemon tea | '' | |
| 22 | 6.9 | - | - | Arrow roots, Matumbo, Plums | White Supote | Rice, Matumbo (offals) | - | Black Beans marsh, Cabbage, Fried Beef, ACVH | '' | |
| 28 | 7.3 | - | - | Black Beans-Marsh, Sausage, Salad (Pineapple, Pawpaw, red Melon) | - | Black Beans-Stew, Hot Lemon water | 4 Plums | Ugali, Kales/Beef stew, Plums, Hot Lemon water | '' | |
| 29 | 6.8 | - | - | Sweet Potatoes, White Supote | 4 Plums | Rice, Beef/Courgettes/Eggplant stew | 2 Plums | Peas-Mukimo (mash), Red Melon, 2 Sweet Bananas ACVH | '' | - |

**April, 2015**

| Date | GI | Pressure | Wt. (Kgs) | Breakfast | Snack 10am | Lunch | Snack 4pm | Dinner | Diabetes Medicine |
|---|---|---|---|---|---|---|---|---|---|
| 3 | 6.4 | 127/72/67 | - | Sweet Potato, Banana | Fried Peas | Rice, Spinach | - | Roast Irish Potato, Amaranthus stew, Fish-Nile Tilapia, Red Melon, ACVH | '' |
| 4 | 7.7 | - | - | Fish-Nile Tilapia, Canned Tomato/Bean Sauce, Arrow roots, Sweet Banana | Plums | Roast Irish Potatoes, Amaranthus, Fish-Nile Tilapia | Banana Crisps, Chocolate Cake | Black Beans-Mukimo, Turkey, Lemon Tea | '' |
| 5 | 6.6 | 129/69/71 | - | Sweet Potatoes, Sweet Bananas | Peas-Fried | Black Beans, Turkey, Cabbage | Sweet Bananas | Amaranthus, Fish-Nile Tilapia, Ugali, Pawpaw Yogurt ACVH | '' |
| 6 | 7.7 | 120/74/71 | - | Carrots /Onion/ Peanut butter/ Marmalade Toast, | Fried Peas | Black Beans, Cabbage Beef stew, Avocado | | Chapati, Lentils, Pawpaw, ACVH | '' |

| Date | GI | Pressure | Wt. (Kgs) | Breakfast | Snack 10am | Lunch | Snack 4pm | Dinner | Diabetes Medicine |
|---|---|---|---|---|---|---|---|---|---|
| | | | | Fish-Nile Perch, 2 Sweet Bananas | | | | | |
| 11 | 7.7 | - | - | Arrow root, Sweet Potatoes/ Egg/Tomatoes fry, Sweet Banana | Tea, Ndazi | - | Rice, Beef/ Cabbage stew, | Beef/Cabbage Stew, Sweet Potatoes, Thorny Melon, ACVH | ' ' |
| 12 | 6.6 | 125/66/73 | - | Toasted Bread, Peas fried | Pop Corns, Banana Crisps | Beef/Cabbage stew | Peas Fried | Local Chicken/Peas-Mukimo, Thorny Melon, ACVH | ' ' |
| 17 | 7 | - | - | Egg, fried Tomatoes, Sausage, Toasted Bread Banana | - | Fish, Beef, Raw/Cooked Vegetables, Fruit Salad | Tea, Snacks | Beef /Cabbage stew, Rice ACVH | ' ' |
| 18 | - | - | 71.3 | Chapati, Kunde, Peas Fried, Pawpaw | | Melon, Sweet Banana | Rice, Kunde, Peas fried | Ugali, African nightshade, RVM | ' ' |
| 19 | 6.1 | - | - | Egg/Tomato/ Chapati Omelet | Pear | Beef/Kales, Ugali, Hot Lemon Water | Sweet Banana | Butter Bean/Maize stew, Kunde, Pear, Hot Lemon water / Honey | ' ' |
| 25 | 6 | - | - | Egg/Fried Tomato, Sausage, Weetabix | - | Boiled Kales, Goat Meat, Peas Mash, RVM | - | Rice, Green gram Stew, Peas fried, ACVH | ' ' |
| 26 | 7.3 | - | | Sweet Potatoes, Peanuts, Pawpaw | Banana Crisps | Rice, Green Gram Stew | - | Butter Bean Mash, Cabbage, Avocado Pear, ACVH | ' ' |

**May,2015**

| Date | GI | Pressure | Wt. (Kgs) | Breakfast | Snack 10am | Lunch | Snack 4pm | Dinner | Diabetes Medicine |
|---|---|---|---|---|---|---|---|---|---|
| 1 | 6.8 | 110/70/72 | - | Carrots/Hoho (Capsicum-bell peppers)/ Onion bread salad Toast, Liver/spleen 2 Sweet Bananas | 2 Sweet Bananas | Butter Bean, Beef/Cabbage stew, Avocado | Green Apple | Chicken, French Beans, Chapati, Pears | No Glucophage |
| 2 | 7.4 | - | - | Sweet Potatoes, Omena, Groundnuts, Sweet Banana | 2 Sweet Bananas | Chicken, French Beans, Chapati, Pawpaw | - | Arrow roots, Cabbage, Peas/Carrots stew, ACVH | ' ' |
| 3 | 6.2 | - | | Chapati, Chicken, Pears | - | Chapati, Chicken, French Beans, Peas, Pawpaw | - | Kales, Rice, Liver, RVM(raw Vegetable Mix) salad | ' ' |
| 9 | 7.3 | 132/75/79 | - | Sweet Potato, Fish-Nile Perch, Pawpaw | - | 2 red Apples, Peas Mash, | - | Kales, Ugali, Pawpaw, ACVH | ' ' |

| | | | | Beef stew | | | | | |
|---|---|---|---|---|---|---|---|---|---|
| 10 | 6.6 | 120/67/75 | - | Egg/Tomato/ Chapati fry, Pawpaw | Big Green Apple | Rice, Matumbo (Offals), Cabbage | ¾ Chapati | Chapati, Chicken, Pawpaw | ' ' |
| 16 | 6.5 | 120/70/76 | - | Arrow roots, Sweet Potato, Catfish, White Supote | | Maize / Beans Stew | Black Forest Cake | Chicken, African nightshade, Ugali ACVH | ' ' |
| 17 | 6.4 | 120/80/79 | - | Omelet – Onion/Tomat oes/egg/ Chapati, White Supote | | Chicken, Ugali, African nightshade , | Beef cutlet, Hot Lemon water | Black Beans Mash, Cabbage/ meat stew, Pawpaw, ACVH | ' ' |
| 23 | 6.3 | 115/64/64 | - | Arrow Roots, Sweet Potatoes, White Supote | Banana | Cashew nuts, Banana crisps | Banana crisps, Cashew nuts,1/4 white Chapati | Catfish, African nightshade, Ugali ,Thorny Melon, ACVH | ' ' |
| 24 | 6.6 | 112/63/73 | - | Arrow Roots, Sweet Potatoes, Catfish, White Supote | Banana crisps, 2 Large Apples | Ugali, Matumbo, African nightshade | White Supote, 2 Large Apples | Maize/ Beans stew, Cabbage/Be ef stew, Thorny Melon, Green tea | ' ' |
| 30 | 6.4 | 105/74/70 | - | Arrow Roots, Catfish, Pawpaw | White chocolat e | Maize/Bea ns stew, French Beans, Avocado, I biscuit | 2 Large Apples | Spinach/Bee f stew, Arrow Roots, Sweet Potatoes, Hot water | ' ' |
| 31 | 6.5 | 124/71/73 | - | Sweet Potatoes, Tilapia Fish stew, White Supote | Banana crisps | Spinach/B eef stew, Arrow Roots, Sweet Potatoes | 2 Sweet Bananas | Chicken, Chapati, pea stews | - |

Note: Exceptional figures highlighted in yellow

# Annex 4: Data on Stage 4(June -December 2015) - No diabetes medication, Glycemic Index above 6mmol/l

| June, 2015 | | | | | | | | | | |
|---|---|---|---|---|---|---|---|---|---|---|
| Date | GI | Pressure | W (Kgs) | Breakfast | Snack 10am | Lunch | Snack 4pm | Dinner | Diabetes Medicine | Remarks |
| 6 | 6.6 | 103/66/77 | - | Arrow roots, Groundnuts , ½ Banana | ½ Banana | Spinach/Be ef Stew, Arrow roots, Sweet Potatoes | - | French Bean Stew, Rice, ½ pear, Yogurt | - | Not taken Glucophage for 2 days |
| 7 | 6.5 | 122/70/73 | - | Sweet Potatoes, Groundnuts , Banana | Mango | French Bean Stew, Rice, Mango | Mango, Passion fruit | Black Beans' Mash, Fried Meat, Avocado, ACVH | - | Relaxed and no work stress |
| 10 | 7.2 | - | - | Fried Meat, Sweet Potatoes, Mango | Tea, Ndazi | Chicken stew, Chapati, Cabbage | ½ Chapati | Roast Irish Potatoes, Fried Beef, Cabbage/ Carrots/O | - | Irregular feeding times Lunch at 3pm |

| Date | GI | Pressure | Wt. (Kgs) | Breakfast | Snack 10am | Lunch | Snack 4pm | Dinner | Diabetes Medicine | Remarks |
|---|---|---|---|---|---|---|---|---|---|---|
| | | | | | | | | nion salad | | Took Asomex-5® |
| 13 | 6.7 | 117/71/74 | - | Chapati/egg /Onion/ Fried Tomato, White Supote | White Supote | Cabbage/Carrots/Irish Potato/Beef stew, Rice, 1 biscuit | Nut chocolate -3 pieces | Roast meat, Black Beans Mash, Avocado, ¼ Orange Fruit, ¼ Pears and Green tea | - | Took Asomex-5® |
| 14 | 7.1 | 143/89/74 | - | Roast meat, Sausage, Sweet Potato, Orange Fruit | White Supote, Purple Passion Fruit | Black Beans Mash, Avocado, Beef/Kales stew, | ½ Orange Fruit | Deep fried Sweet Potato, Arrow roots, Green tea | - | Restless Night<br><br>Sleepless Night in a smelly newly painted room |
| 20 | - | - | - | Small amounts of Rice crisps, Arrow roots, Roast Irish Potatoes, Bacon, Sausage, red Melon, Pineapple | | Chicken, Beans, Groundnuts, Red Melon, Banana, Tangerine | - | Rice, Beef/Lentils stew, Tangerine | - | Visiting the coastal area |
| 21 | 6.3 | 139/80/71 | - | Bread/egg fry/ Tangerine | - | Fruits- Tangerine, Banana, red Melon | - | Rice, Beef/Lentils stew, Tangerine | - | Relaxed mood- sorted out an office matter |
| 27 | 6.2 | 135/77/75 | - | Cassava, Groundnuts, Cashew nuts, Sweet Potato | Banana | Rice, Beef/Green grams stew, 1 Ginger biscuit | Catfish | Catfish, Spinach, Ugali, Thorny Melon, ACVH | - | Relaxed mood-In a workshop |
| 28 | 6.7 | 106/61/68 | - | Sweet Potatoes, Groundnuts, Cashew nuts, Orange Fruit | Peas, 2 Ginger biscuits | Chicken curry, Chapati, hot Lemon water | - | Green Peas /Maize Mash, Beef/ Cabbage stew, Thorny Melon, ACVH | - | - |

**July, 2015**

| Date | GI | Pressure | Wt. (Kgs) | Breakfast | Snack 10am | Lunch | Snack 4pm | Dinner | Diabetes Medicine | Remarks |
|---|---|---|---|---|---|---|---|---|---|---|
| 4 | 7.3 | 116/64/74 | - | Onion/Tomato, Oats bread with Margarine, Pawpaw, Purple Passion fruit | Tea/cake | Fish, Chicken, Beef, roast Potatoes, Red Melon, Pawpaw, cake | - | Eggplant/ Cauliflower/ Beef stew, Purple Passion fruit, ACVH | - | Changed exercise from dancing to acrobats Overeating, eating of sugary foods<br><br>Took Asomex-5® |
| 5 | 6.7 | 122/76/70 | - | Rye bread, Sweet Potato, Large | - | Chicken, Roasted Irish | - | Spinach, Eggplant/ Cauliflow | - | - |

| Date | GI | Pressure | Wt. (Kgs) | Breakfast | Snack 10am | Lunch | Snack 4pm | Dinner | Diabetes Medicine | Remarks |
|---|---|---|---|---|---|---|---|---|---|---|
| | | | | Apple | | Potatoes, Spinach, Hot Lemon water | | er, red Melon, ACVH | | |
| 11 | 6.7 | 106/59/68 | - | Sweet Potatoes, Fish-Tilapia Red Melon, Tree Tomato fruit, Juice-Avocado/Banana | Banana | Fish-Tilapia-deep fried, Roast Potatoes | Tea/Sausage | Fish-Nile perch, African nightshade, Ugali | - | Took Asomex-5® |
| 12 | 6.4 | 116/58/66 | - | Toasted sandwich-Oats bread/ Onions/ Carrots, Fish Nile perch, Tree Tomato fruit | | African nightshade, Ugali, Fish-Nile perch, Pear | Macadamia(Queensland ) Nuts, Cashew nuts, Groundnuts | Mash-Maize/Beans/Pumpkin leaves, Cabbage/ meat /Pumpkin stew, Mango, *Mursik* | | Took Asomex-5® |
| 18 | 6.8 | 118/65/73 | - | Arrow roots, Fish-Trout, Pawpaw | Homemade Orange Fruit juice | Cabbage/ Beef stew, Banana/ Sweet Potato Mash | - | Ugali, Kales/Beef stew, Pawpaw, ACVH | - | Took Asomex-5® |
| 19 | 6.7 | 121/73/73 | - | Omelet, Fish-Tilapia-deep fried, White Supote fruit, Lemonade | - | Avocado / Pawpaw salad | 2 slices of bread /egg toast, Hot Lemon water | Chapati, Cabbage/ Beef stew, Kales, Hot Lemon water | - | - |
| 25 | 4.7 | 116/74/72 | - | Onion/egg/ Fried Tomato, Oats bread, Pawpaw | Mango, Banana crisps | Chicken curry, Chapati, Hot Lemon water | - | Plain yogurt, ½ Mango, ½ Thorny Melon | - | Fruit/Yogurt dinner |
| 26 | 6.3 | 106/64/72 | - | Oats bread with Margarine, Fish- Tilapia soup | Banana | Roast Chicken, Roast Irish Potatoes, Spinach/ Carrots, Hot Lemon water | - | Maize/Beans (Githeri) Stew. Avocado, Mango, Plain Yogurt | - | - |

**August , 2015**

| Date | GI | Pressure | Wt. (Kgs) | Breakfast | Snack 10am | Lunch | Snack 4pm | Dinner | Diabetes Medicine | Remarks |
|---|---|---|---|---|---|---|---|---|---|---|
| 1 | 6.3 | 127/74/71 | 71.9 | Sweet Potatoes, Fish Tilapia, Mango | Mango – small size | Maize/Beans/Beef/ Cabbage stew, Hot Lemon water | 5 loquats, | Ugali, Fish-Tilapia, Kales, Thorny Melon, yogurt 100mls | - | - |
| 2 | 6.1 | - | - | Oats meal, Groundnuts, Cashew nuts, Pawpaw | - | Chicken curry, Chapati, Hot Lemon water | 2 loquats, | Chicken/Peas stew, Kales, 1 slice of bread, Pawpaw, ACVH | - | Oats, Chicken, light meals<br><br>Pressure machine out of order |

| Date | GI | Pressure | Wt. (Kgs) | Breakfast | Snack 10am | Lunch | Snack 4pm | Dinner | Diabetes Medicine | Remarks |
|---|---|---|---|---|---|---|---|---|---|---|
| 8 | 6.9 | 114/69/66 | - | arrow roots, Fried egg, ½ Mango | A lot of Banana crisps, Ginger biscuits, | - | - | Chapati, Green grams/Beef stew, Thorny Melon, Tangerine | - | No lunch, Dinner at 9.45pm-irregular feeding<br><br>Have a cold, attended a friends funeral |
| 9 | 6.9 | - | - | Arrow roots, Fish -Nile perch, ½ Mango | 2 Sweet Bananas, ½ Mango | Beef/Green gram stew, Cabbage, Chapati, | - | A lot of Peas/Maize Mash, Cabbage, Fish Nile perch, Thorny Melon, Cold water | - | Sweet fruits, Overeating<br><br>Pressure machine out of order |
| 14 | 6.1 | - | - | Arrow roots, Sweet Potatoes, Irish Potatoes, Cashew nuts | Passion juice, Sweet Bananas | Chicken, Cabbage, Kales, 2 big size Sweet Banana | - | Mala( Fermented milk) 250 mls, Pawpaw big portion | - | Light meals, Chicken<br><br>Pynstop®-prescriptio n to replace Asomex-5® |
| 15 | 6.4 | 104/64/65 | - | Arrow roots, Almond nuts, Banana | - | Rice, Beef /Cabbage stew | - | Ugali, Kales/Beef stew, Pawpaw | - | - |
| 24 | 6.2 | - | - | - | - | - | - | - | - | Been to a neighborin g country throughout the week |
| 29 | 6 | 114/65/64 | - | Arrow roots, Sweet Potatoes, Chicken Sausage, Pawpaw | 2 small Mandazi | Beans/Ma ize Mash, ½ big Avocado | - | Ugali, Beef/Kales/ Spinach stew, Pawpaw, ACVH | - | On leave-relaxed at home |
| 30 | 6.3 | 104/62/71 | - | Arrow roots, 2 small Mandazi, Chicken Sausage, Pawpaw | 2 small Mandazi | Rice, Beef/Kale s stew, Pawpaw | 2 Passion fruits | Rice, Spinach, liver, \Melon | - | Have a cold-taken Piriton |

September, 2015

| Date | GI | Pressure | Wt. (Kgs) | Breakfast | Snack 10am | Lunch | Snack 4pm | Dinner | Diabetes Medicine | Remarks |
|---|---|---|---|---|---|---|---|---|---|---|
| 5 | 6.3 | 130/72/66 | - | Fried egg, 2 slices Oats bread, Pawpaw | Passion juice | Roasted Goat meat, 3 slices Oats bread | Ginger tea, egg omelet, Sweet Potato | Ugali, Beef/Kales stew, Pawpaw | - | - |
| 6 | 6 | 130/63/68 | 72.2 | Small portion of Sweet Potatoes, toasted Oats bread/Margari ne/Peanut butter/Onion/ Carrots, Mango small size | 1 Passion fruit | Ugali, Beef/Kal es stew | - | Chicken, Spinach, Lentils, ½ Chapati, ¼ Orange Fruit | - | Light meals, Chicken<br><br>Changed cooking oil to cooking fat |
| 12 | 7.4 | 109/65/69 | - | Toasted Oats bread/Onion/C arrots , Cashew nuts, | - | - | Fish-Nile perch, Chapati, | Beef/Broccol i/French Beans stew, 1/3 roasted | - | Irregular eating, missing lunch |

| Date | GI | Pressure | Wt. (Kgs) | Breakfast | Snack 10am | Lunch | Snack 4pm | Dinner | Diabetes Medicine | Remarks |
|---|---|---|---|---|---|---|---|---|---|---|
| | | | | Peanuts, Almond nuts, Pawpaw | | | Hot Lemon water | Maize cob, Red Melon | | Dinner- 10 pm<br><br>In meetings all day |
| 19 | 6.3 | 120/66/73 | - | Arrow roots, Sweet Potato, Catfish, Banana | Green Apple | Maize/Beans, Beef/Kales/Cabbage stew | - | Beef stew, Lugwarts, Red Melon | - | - |
| 20 | - | - | - | Sweet Potatoes, Almond nuts, Pawpaw | - | Fried Beef, Peas/Cabbage stew, fried Black Beans | - | - | - | In a party- avoided carbohydrate which were all white starch |
| 26 | 6.3 | 121/70/72 | - | Arrow roots, Catfish, Passion fruit | 2 Sweet Bananas, 1 big Banana | Maize/Beans/ Beef/Cabbage/ Kales stew | 2 Lugwarts | Green Banana/ Potato/meat stew, Spinach, Pawpaw | - | Morning snacks at 10 and 11 am |
| 27 | 6.4 | 125/74/71 | - | Toasted Oats bread/Onion/ Carrots sandwich, Pawpaw | Banana crisps, Lugwarts | Green Banana/Irish Potato, Beef/Spinach stew, | - | Maize/Beans, Beef/Cabbage stew, Melon | - | - |

October,2015

| Date | GI | Pressure | Wt. (Kgs) | Breakfast | Snack 10am | Lunch | Snack 4pm | Dinner | Diabetes Medicine | Remarks |
|---|---|---|---|---|---|---|---|---|---|---|
| 3 | 6.8 | 117/62/71 | - | 2 toasts, 2 eggs, 2 Sausages, Fruit salad(Pawpaw, red Melon, Pineapple, Banana) | Tea, Arrow root - small portion | Fish, Cabbage salad, Kales, Beef stew, 1 piece each of- Banana & Melon | Tea, Black Forest Cake | Ugali, Meat/Kales stew, Pawpaw | - | In a workshop |
| 4 | 6.8 | 123/62/65 | - | Oats-1/2 cup, Boiled Catfish, Pawpaw | 5 small Lugwarts, Passion fruit | Maize/Beans stew, Kales, Avocado ½ piece | 3 Ginger biscuits | Chicken, cowpea leaves, ½ Chapati | - | Dinner at 11.30pm |
| 10 | 6.8 | 125/62/63 | - | Sweet Potatoes, Almond nuts, Groundnuts, Pawpaw, Lugwarts | Whole Banana | Rice, Beef/Cabbage stew, 1 Ginger biscuit | Roasted Maize small piece, 1 Sweet Banana | Green Peas/Maize Mash, Beef/Cabbage stew, Thorny Melon, Fish soup | - | Overate dinner |
| 11 | 6.5 | 115/64/68 | - | Toasted Oats bread/Carrots/ Onion sandwich, Boiled Catfish, Red water Melon | 5 tree Strawberry fruits, 6 Lugwarts, | Green Peas/Maize Mash, Spinach | - | Ugali, cowpea leaves,, Spinach, Deep fried Catfish, Fish soup, Thorny Melon | - | - |
| 17 | 6.7 | 127/71/70 | - | Toasted Oats bread/Carrots/ Onion sandwich, | ½ Green Apple, Meat Samosa | Fried Goat meat, Maize/Irish | 2 tree Strawberry fruits, 2 Lugwarts | Salad - Pawpaw/ Mango | - | Goat meat highly salted |

| Date | GI | Pressure | Wt. (Kgs) | Breakfast | Snack 10am | Lunch | Snack 4pm | Dinner | Diabetes Medicine | Remarks |
|---|---|---|---|---|---|---|---|---|---|---|
|  |  |  |  | Almond nuts, Groundnuts, Pawpaw, 6 tree Strawberry fruits |  | Potato/Pumpkin leaves Mash |  |  |  |  |
| 18 | 6.3 | 120/70/69 | - | Toasted Oats bread with Margarine, Catfish, Pawpaw | Tree Strawberry fruits, Pawpaw | Chapati, Beef/Cabbage stew, | - | Butter Beans/Maize stew, Cabbage/Beef stew, Avocado, Thorny Melon, Fish soup | - | - |
| 24 | 6.6 | 118/70/71 | 71.1 | Spanish omelet, Black Beans, Sweet Potato, Pineapple | Banana crisps | Chapati, Beef/Cabbage, cow Peas | - | Sweet Potatoes, Beef/Cauliflower/Carrots stew, Passion fruit | - | In a workshop |
| 25 | 6.4 | 134/73/71 | - | Sweet Potato, Almond nuts, Groundnuts, Passion fruit | 2 Sweet Bananas | Sweet Potatoes, Cauliflower/Beef, Carrots stew, | 1 Sweet Banana | Chapati, Peas/Beef stew, Melon | - | A lot of office work carried home |
| 31 | 6.1 | 136/71/68 | - | Sweet Potato, Arrow Roots, Beans, Beef Sausage, Pineapple | Banana | Maize/Potato/Greens Mash, Deep fried Chicken, Cabbage, Beef soup | - | Kidney/African nightshade, fruit salad-Pawpaw/Banana/Melon | - | In a workshop -26th -30th |

November, 2015

| Date | GI | Pressure | Wt. (Kgs) | Breakfast | Snack 10am | Lunch | Snack 4pm | Dinner | Diabetes Medicine | Remarks |
|---|---|---|---|---|---|---|---|---|---|---|
| 1 | 6.4 | 124/67/74 | - | Linseed coated Margarine bread, Fruit salad-Banana/Pawpaw/Melon | Fruit salad-Banana/Pawpaw/Melon | Ugali, Cattle Kidney, African nightshade leaves, 2 Passion fruits | - | Maize/Pigeon Peas, Peas Mash, Beef/Cabbage stew, Thorny Melon | - | - |
| 7 | 6.4 | 123/69/72 | - | Sweet Potato, Fish- Nile perch, Pawpaw | Banana | Maize/Pigeon Peas, Peas Mash, Beef/Cabbage stew, | - | Chapati, Chicken, Peas/Carrots stew, ½ Tangerine | - | - |
| 8 | 7.0 | 139/73/73 | - | ½ Chapati, Egg/Tomato/Onion fry | Passion fruit/1/4 Mango | Chapati, Chicken, Spinach, Passion fruit | - | Butter Beans/Maize stew, Beef/Cabbage stew, Pawpaw | - | Irregular meal times<br><br>Lunch 3 pm |
| 14 | 6.8 | - | - | Lima Beans/Maize Mash, Chicken, Pawpaw | Ndazi, Beef Sausage, Samosa, Tea, 1 big Apple | - | Banana crisps, Groundnuts | Ugali, Fish-common carp, African nightshade leaves, Thorny Melon, Pawpaw, ¼ Orange Fruit | - | Inadequate sleep<br><br>Slept at 1am |
| 15 | 7.7 | 128/71/71 | - | Toasted | - | Ugali, | ½ Mango | Maize/Beans | - | Inadequa |

| Date | GI | Pressure | Wt. (kgs) | Breakfast | Snack 10am | Lunch | Snack 4pm | Dinner | Diabetes Medicine | Remarks |
|---|---|---|---|---|---|---|---|---|---|---|
| | | | | bread /Carrots/ Onion/ sandwich, Boiled egg, Pawpaw/or ang salad | | Fish-common carp, African nightshade | | stew, Beef/Cabbag e stew, Avocado, Thorny Melon | | te sleep<br><br>Slept at 2 am-working on office carry over work |
| 21 | 6.9 | 123/72/73 | - | ½ Chapati, Fried egg, Pawpaw | - | Butter Beans/Mai ze Mash, Beef/Cabb age stew | Apple | Sweet Potatoes, Beef/ Cauliflower stew | - | - |
| 22 | 6.6 | 127/76/70 | - | Sweet Potatoes, Catfish | Pawpaw | Maize/Bea ns stew, Beef/Kale s stew, Pawpaw | 1 Ginger biscuit Beef cutlet, tea | Fish soup, Pawpaw | - | Consume d Beef cutlet at 7pm |
| 28 | 6.1 | 130/68/67 | - | Toasted Oats bread/ Onion/ Carrots sandwich, Almond nuts, Groundnuts , Pawpaw | Banana | Arrow roots, Beef/ Cauliflow er/ Carrots stew | - | Ugali, Fish-deep fried/Onion/ Carrots fried, African nightshade Greens, Pawpaw | - | Low sugar feeds |
| 29 | 6.8 | 120/70/71 | - | Sweet Potatoes, Arrow Roots, Groundnuts , Pawpaw | 1 Sweet Banana | Fish soup, Ugali, Fish-deep fried Catfish,, African shade Greens, | 1 big Sweet Banana, Banana crisps | A lot of butter Beans/Maize stew, Beef/ Cauliflower/ Broccoli/ Parsley/ Courgettes stew | - | - |



| Date | GI | Pressure | Wt. (kgs) | Breakfast | Snack 10am | Lunch | Snack 4pm | Dinner | Diabetes Medicine | Remarks |
|---|---|---|---|---|---|---|---|---|---|---|
| 5 | 6.6 | 132/69/69 | - | Spanish omelet, Toasted bread | Ginger tea, Scone(Ca ke) | Noodles, Broiler Chicken, boiled Goat meat, Cabbage, RVM, Pineapple, Water Melon | Black tea, Sweet chocolate cake | Butter Bean/Maize/ Irish Potato stew, Pawpaw | - | In a workshop. Had a headache, suspected Ginger tea for headache |
| 6 | 6.3 | 126/71/70 | 71.1 | Butter Bean/Maiz e/Irish Potato stew, African nightshade Greens, Pawpaw | 1 Sweet Ndazi | Meat stew, Cabbage | Processe d Passion juice-100mls | Chapati, Offals/Spina ch stew, Pawpaw | - | - |
| 12 | 6.8 | 123/68/60 | - | Sweet Potatoes, Fish-Tilapia, Pawpaw | Big Mango, Banana | Rice, Beef/lentil s stew, Banana crisps | - | Butter Beans/Maize stew, Beef/Cabbag e stew, Avocado/Ba nana milk shake | - | - |
| 12 | 6.5 | 130/68/71 | - | Sweet Potatoes, Fish- deep fried Tilapia, Pawpaw | 2 Passion fruits | Butter Beans/Mai ze stew, Beef/Cabb age stew, Avocado/ | ½ Chapati | Chapati, Chicken, Peas/Carrots stew, Melon | - | - |

| Date | GI | Pressure | Wt. (kgs) | Breakfast | Snack 10am | Lunch | Snack 4pm | Dinner | Diabetes Medicine | Remarks |
|---|---|---|---|---|---|---|---|---|---|---|
| | | | | | | Banana milk shake | | | | |
| 19 | 6.5 | 124/72/67 | - | Sweet Potatoes, small pieces of Sweet Lemon cake & Black forest cake, Catfish, 2 Plums | 1 Banana | Rice, minced meat, Cabbage, 1 Ginger biscuit | 3 big Plums, 1 slice of Oats bread with Margarine spread | Sweet Potatoes, Beef/ Cauliflower/ Courgettes/ Broccoli stew, big piece of Pawpaw | - | Oats bread at 7pm |
| 20 | 6.3 | 131/72/74 | 71.1 | Toasted Oats bread/Carrots/ Onion sandwich, Catfish, 2 Plums | 2 Plums, Piece of Carrot | Sweet Potatoes, Beef/ Cauliflower/ Courgettes, Broccoli/Carrots stew | ½ Banana | Butter Beans/Maize stew, Beef/Cabbage/Butternut Pumpkin, Avocado/ Banana juice | - | - |
| 26 | 6.6 | 131/71/72 | 71.1 | Bread, Lemon cake, Roasted Goat meat, ¼ Orange Fruit | 3 Plums | 1/4 White floor Chapati, 4 big pieces of French fries, Samosa, Chicken, Tilapia, Beef/Carrots stew, Kebab, Avocado | Pawpaw, Pineapple, Lemon cake, kebab | 1 Sweet Banana, cup of Lemon Green tea | - | - |
| 27 | 7.1 | 132/78/68 | - | Ndazi, Samosa, Broiler Chicken, ½ Orange Fruit | - | Ugali, RVM, Fish-Tilapia, | Tree Tomato, 2 Plums | Butter Bean/Maize stew, Beef/Spinach, Kales, Avocado, Thorny Melon | - | Inadequate rest<br><br>Had a headache and a restless Night, took a Piriton |

Note: Exceptional figures highlighted in yellow

## Annex 5- Stage 5(January to May 2016): No diabetes medication – GI less than 6mmol/l

| January, 2016 | | | | | | | | | | |
|---|---|---|---|---|---|---|---|---|---|---|
| Date | GI | Pressure | Wt. (kgs) | Breakfast | Snack 10am | Lunch | Snack 4pm | Dinner | Diabetes Medicine | Remarks |
| 2 | 6.0 | 126/72/67 | 71.9 | Sweet Potatoes, Almond nuts, Groundnuts, 2 Plums | 2 Plums | Chapati, Chicken, Peas/Irish Potato/ Carrots stew, fruit salad-Bananas, Pawpaw, Pineapple, Orange | ½ Chapati | fruit salad-Bananas, Pawpaw, Pineapple, Orange Fruit, Passion in plain yogurt | - | On leave up to 1st February, Changed Exercise from acrobats to athletics Good rest, light dinner, Chicken, |

| | | | | | | | | | | |
|---|---|---|---|---|---|---|---|---|---|---|
| | | | | | | Fruit, Passion in plain yogurt | | | | Peas<br><br>Spent a restful, happy day with friends and family |
| 3 | 6.4 | 135/73/69 | - | ½ Chapati, Almond nuts, Groundnuts, 2 Plums, 1 small white Supote | 2 Plums | Sweet Potatoes, Peas/Irish Potatoes /Carrots stew | 2 Plums | Maize/Beans stew, Beef/Kales stew, Pineapple, Fish soup | - | - |
| 9 | 5.5 | 150/78/72 | 72 | Nuts(Almonds, Groundnuts, Cashew), 2 slices toasted bread, 1 Chicken Sausage, 2 Plums | 1 small white Supote | Beef/Kales stew, Lentils, Rice, ½ Lemon in a glass of water | Nuts(Groundnuts, Cashew), Popcorn, 1 slice Oats bread with Margarine | Offals, Arrow Roots, Courgettes/ Cauliflower /Broccoli stew | - | Nuts, Chicken Sausage, Lentils could have contributed to low sugar level?<br><br>Taken Nuts throughout the week. High blood pressure due to excitement of reduced glucose reading |
| 10 | 5.2 | 145/71/71 | - | Nuts (Almonds, Groundnuts, Cashew), 2 slices toasted bread, 1 Chicken Sausage, ½ Mango | 1 Sweet Banana | Offals, Arrow Roots, Courgettes/ Cauliflower / Broccoli stew, , ½ Lemon in a glass of water | - | Beef/Kales stew, Black Beans Mash, piece of Pineapple | - | Nuts, Chicken Sausage? Type of Vegetables |
| 16 | 4.7 | 130/70/74 | 70.8 | Nuts (Almonds, Groundnuts, Cashew), Beef/Black Beans stew, Avocado, Chicken Sausage, 2 Plums | 2 Plums | Beef/ Spinach/ Kales stew, Ugali, 1 Plums | 2 Plums, piece of Pawpaw | Beef/Irish Potato /Green Peas stew, Rice, 2 Plums | - | Nuts, Chicken Sausage?<br><br>On atorvastatin 10mg since 13th to reduce triglycerides from desired 1.71 mmol/L to current 3.65, Also remedy to pulsating head veins?. Reduced salt and cooking fat |
| 17 | 5.4 | 132/78/70 | - | Nuts (Almonds, Groundnuts, Cashew), Beef/ Peas/Irish Potato stew, Rice, 2 | 2 Plums | Black Beans/ Maize Mash, Beef/ Kales/ Spinach stew | 4 Plums, Pawpaw, ½ Chapati | Beef/Lentils stew, ½ Chapati, 2 Plums | - | Nuts? Leave?<br><br>Chapati snack at 7pm and not 6 pm<br><br>atorvastatin 10mg |

| Date | GI | Pressure | Wt. (Kgs) | Breakfast | Snack 10am | Lunch | Snack 4pm | Dinner | Diabetes Medicine | Remarks |
|---|---|---|---|---|---|---|---|---|---|---|
| | | | | Plums | | | | | | |
| 23 | 5.0 | 124/69/70 | 71.3 | Nuts (Almonds, Groundnuts, Cashew), Sweet Potatoes, Pawpaw | ½ Banana | Butter Beans/ Beef/ Pumpkin stew, Amaranthus | Black Forest Cake sprinkled with Lemon juice pressed directly from a Lemon | Beef/ Cabbage/ Carrots stew, pasta, Pawpaw covered with plain yogurt | - | Nuts? Leave?<br><br>atorvastatin 10mg |
| 24 | 4.9 | 122/70/71 | - | ½ Chapati Pawpaw Nuts (Almonds, Groundnuts, Cashew) | Pawpaw | Amaranthus, Butternut /Beans/ Maize stew | Pawpaw, Purple Passion fruit | Chicken broiler, Potato/ Green Banana Mash, plain yogurt | | Nuts? Leave?<br><br>atorvastatin 10mg |
| 30 | 5.2 | 132/70/72 | 71.5 | Sweet Potato, Pawpaw, Nuts (Almonds, Groundnuts, Cashew) | - | Rice, Beef/ Cabbage stew | Tea | Beans/ Maize/Broccoli/ Courgettes/ Capsicum stew, Pawpaw | - | Nuts? Leave? |
| 31 | 5.4 | 121/71/63 | - | Pawpaw, slices of toasted Oats bread, handful of Nuts(Almonds, Groundnuts, Cashew) | Nuts (Almonds, Groundnuts, Cashew) | Maize/Beans/ Beef stew, Courgettes, red Capsicum, Pineapple | Tea | ½ Chapati, Beef/ Courgettes/ Capsicum/ Broccoli/ Green Peas/Butter Nut Stew, Pawpaw | - | Nuts? Leave? |

**February, 2016**

| Date | GI | Pressure | Wt. (Kgs) | Breakfast | Snack 10am | Lunch | Snack 4pm | Dinner | Diabetes Medicine | Remarks |
|---|---|---|---|---|---|---|---|---|---|---|
| 6 | 6.1 | 130/73/68 | 71 | Roasted Bananas, Sweet Potatoes, Nuts (Almonds, Groundnuts, Cashew& walnuts) | 2 Plums | Tilapia, Maize/ Beans/ Irish Potatoes Mash/ Pumpkin stew | I Plums, 2 small Mandazi | Beef/ Cauliflower/ Broccoli/ Courgettes stew, Thorny Melon | - | Resumed duty on 1st |
| 7 | 5.5 | 123/74/73 | - | Toasted Oats/linseed breed, ¼ Mango | 2 Plums | Sweet Potato, Beef/ Cauliflower/Broccoli, Courgettes/ Carrots stew | 2 Plums, ¼ Mango | Green Peas/Irish Potatoes/ Green Bananas Mash, Kales, Thorny Melon | - | Regular meals and timings |
| 13 | 5.7 | 132/71/70 | 69.5 | Sweet Potatoes, Nuts (Almonds, Groundnuts, Cashew& walnuts), ¼ Mango, 1 white Supote | 3 Plums | Brown Rice, Beef/French Beans/Spinach stew | 1 Plums | Fruit salad (Pawpaw/ Banana/ zebra Melon) mixed with plain Yogurt | - | Took lunch at 3pm ( irregular meals), Replacing dinner with just fruit salad |
| 14 | 6.2 | 120/72/70 | - | 2 slices Oats/linseed toasted bread, ½ Banana | 2 Plums | Rice, French Beans/ Cabbage stew, 1 Plum | 2 Plums | 1/2/Chapati, Beef/ Chicken, Beef/Peas stew, ¼ | - | Dinner at 10.20pm ( irregular meal), started |

| Date | GI | Pressure | Wt. (Kgs) | Breakfast | Snack 10am | Lunch | Snack 4pm | Dinner | Diabetes Medicine | Possible Explanation To GI Reading |
|---|---|---|---|---|---|---|---|---|---|---|
| | | | | | | | | Mango | | missing Beef in some meals |
| 20 | 5.7 | 135/69/73 | 68.9 | Arrow Roots, Nuts (Almonds, Groundnuts, Cashew& walnuts), | 1 big Plums | Rice, African nightshade vegetables,1/2 Ginger biscuit | 3 Plums | Fruit salad ( Pineapple/ Thorny Melon) in 2 table spoons of plain Yogurt | - | Stressful Night |
| 21 | 5.0 | 125/65/71 | - | 2 slices Oats/ linseed toasted bread, 1 Ndazi, 2 Plums | 1 Plums | Sweet Potatoes, Goat meat/ Cauliflower/ yellow Capsicum/ Courgettes/ Butternut stew, | Ground nuts | Maize/ Beans/Pum pkin leaves Mash, Goat meat/ Cabbage stew, piece of Pineapple, ½ Thorny Melon | - | Type of vegetables<br><br>Busy day, regular meals |
| 27 | 5.6 | 127/68/67 | 69.2 | Sweet Potatoes, Nuts (Almond, Groundnut) | 1 large Banana | Rice, African nightshade and Kales vegetables, Offals | 3 Plums | Irish Potatoes, Goat meat/ Cabbage stew,1/4 Mango | - | - |
| 28 | 5.7 | 125/67/69 | - | 2 slices Oats/ linseed toasted bread, ½ Banana, ¼ Mango | 2 Plums, whole fruit process ed Orange Fruit juice | Brown Ugali, Cabbage, fried Goat meat | 2 Plums | ¼ Chapati, Goat meat/Green Peas/ butternut/ Irish Potato stew | - | Late lunch-3pm |
| **March, 2016** | | | | | | | | | | |
| Date | GI | Pressure | Wt. (Kgs) | Breakfast | Snack 10am | Lunch | Snack 4pm | Dinner | Diabetes Medicine | Possible Explanation To GI Reading |
| 5 | 5.2 | 124/74/69 | 68.9 | Arrow Roots, white Supote, Nuts (Almond, Groundnut) . Mango | 1 Plums | Brown Rice, Goat meat/Cabbag e/ Pumpkin stew,1 Ginger biscuit | 5 Groundn uts | Brown Ugali, Goat meat/cow pea(Kunde) leaves stew, white Supote/Plu ms | - | Nuts? |
| 6 | - | 120/65/69 | - | 2 slices Oats/linsee d toasted bread, 1 Plums, 1 white Supote | 1 Plums | Brown Ugali, Goat meat/African Blackshade/ Cabbage stew, white Supote | 1 Plums | Irish Potatoes, Goat meat/ Pumpkin/ butter Beans stew, large piece of Pineapple | - | Fruits taken after food |
| 12 | 5.7 | 125/67/69 | 68.9 | Nuts ( Almonds, Groundnuts and macadamia ), 1 white Supote | 2 Plums | Brown Rice, Peas stew, 1 Ginger biscuit | 1 slice of Oats/ linseed bread | Brown Ugali, Kales, piece of zebra Melon | - | - |
| 13 | 5.8 | 127/71/69 | - | 2 slices Oats/linsee d toasted bread, 1 white Supote | 2 Plums | Brown Rice, Beef/Cauliflo wer/Broccoli /Kales stew, 1 Plums | 2 Plums | Maize/Peas /Green Bananas/Iri sh Potato Mash, Beef/Spina ch stew | - | - |
| 19 | 5.7 | 130/73/71 | 69 | Arrow Roots, | 2 Plums | Nile perch Fish fillet, | - | Fruit (Banana, | - | Hotel food. Late lunch |

| | | | | Mango | | French flies, fresh Melon/ Mango juice | | Pawpaw, Pears) salad in plain Yogurt | | |
|---|---|---|---|---|---|---|---|---|---|---|
| 20 | 6.0 | 127/71/78 | - | 2 slices Oats/ linseed toasted bread, Mango | - | Rice, French Beans stew, Plums | - | Maize/Black Beans (Njahi)/ Green Banana/ Irish Potato Mash, | - | Late lunch |
| 26 | 5.8 | 130/69/69 | 68.6 | 2 slices Oats/ linseed toasted bread, ½ Thorny Melon | Piece of Mango | ½ Chapati, local Chicken/Peas stew | - | ½ Chapati, local Chicken/Peas stew | - | - |
| 27 | 5.3 | 128/68/72 | - | Sweet Potato, Mango fruit | Mango | Chapati, Sweet Potato, local Chicken/Peas stew, Thorny Melon | - | Fruit salad ( Sweet Banana/ Mango/ Thorny Melon) in Yogurt | - | Chicken/ Peas |



| Date | GI | Pressure | Wt. (Kgs) | Breakfast | Snack 10am | Lunch | Snack 4pm | Dinner | Diabetes Medicine | Remarks |
|---|---|---|---|---|---|---|---|---|---|---|
| 2 | 5.8 | 130/69/73 | 68.6 | Sweet Potatoes, white Supote | white Supote, big Ndazi, Sausage | Rice, Cabbage | - | Roast Goat meat, Chapati, vegetable – salad (Tomatoes/ Onions/ Parsley) | - | Irregular meals, overeating |
| 3 | 5.7 | 129/71/70 | - | Roast Goat meat, 1/2/ Chapati, Mango | - | Goat meat/Lentils/ Carrots stew, Chapati | Roast Goat meat | Maize Beans stew, cow pea leaves vegetables. Melon | - | - |
| 9 | 5.3 | 131/72/64 | 68.2 | Fried egg, 2 slices of toasted bread | porridge | Broiler Chicken , Kales, Chapati from sifted white floor | Fish | Fermented milk, Thorny Melon, Mango | - | Late dinner-10pm |
| 10 | 5.3 | 129/66/66 | - | Sweet Potatoes, Mango | - | Brown Ugali, Fish, Kales | Fish | Goat meat/butter Beans/ butternut stew, Pineapple | - | |
| 16 | 5.3 | 129/68/67 | 68 | 2 slices of bread, deep fried Fish, Pawpaw | ½ Banana | Broiler Chicken, 1/2/ Chapati from white sifted wheat flour, Cabbage, zebra Melon | processed Passion juice | Deep fried Fish, vegetable salad, brown Ugali, ¼ Pears | - | - |
| 17 | 6.1 | 127/71/72 | - | 2 slices of toasted bread, boiled Fish, ½ Banana | ¼ Pears | Brown Ugali, Kales/Cabbage | ½ Chapati | Goat meat/Green Peas/ butternut, Spinach, ½ Chapati | - | - |
| 23 | 5.7 | 133/69/68 | 67.8 | - | - | - | - | - | - | - |



| Date | GI | Pressure | Wt. (Kgs) | Breakfast | Snack 10am | Lunch | Snack 4pm | Dinner | Diabetes Medicine | Remarks |
|---|---|---|---|---|---|---|---|---|---|---|
| 1 | 6.0 | 133/72/63 | 68.1 | Sweet Potatoes, | Purple Passion | Beef/ Cabbage | Pears | Deep fried Chicken, | - | Irregular meals, missed |

| | | | | Nuts (Almond, Groundnut), Pawpaw | fruit | stew, brown Rice, white Onion | | Beef/Butter nut Stew, Cabbage, Green Peas, ½ Chapati | | exercise for 2 weeks, attended a workshop, attended burial of a close relative |
|---|---|---|---|---|---|---|---|---|---|---|
| 7 | 5.2 | 138/71/70 | 68.5 | ½ Chapati, ½ Avocado, ½ Banana | ½ Banana, 1 boiled egg, 10 pieces of French fries | Beef/cow pea leaves vegetables stew, Cabbage, Chapati | - | Brown Ugali, African nightshade vegetables, zebra Melon | - | Happy-Organized a successful agricultural show |
| 21 | 5.4 | 137/77/70 | 67.3 | - | - | - | - | - | - | - |
| 22 | 6.0 | 125/65/64 | - | - | - | - | - | - | - | - |
| 28 | 5.6 | 120/64/56 | 67.9 | Sweet Potatoes, Orange Fruit, tree straw berries | Beef/ Kales stew, Maize, Beans, Irish Potatoes/ Green Bananas Mash, | - | Chicken, Chapati, Green Peas/ Carrots stew | - | - | Took dinner at 11pm- irregular meals |

Note: Exceptional figures highlighted in yellow

## Annex 6: Some common food and simple methods used to prepare them

| S/NO | Food/Drink | Constituents | Preparation | Remarks |
|---|---|---|---|---|
| 1 | Tea | Whole Cow's milk, Tea Leaves, Water, | Milk +water (1:2) + tea leaves to required color, boil, stir and continue boiling for 5 more minutes and sieve. Mix a teaspoonful of soya Bean flour with a cup of tea and consume while hot | Tea is taken twice daily at 7am in the morning (can be an hour earlier or later), and at 6pm ( can be an hour earlier or later) |
| 2 | Chapati | Brown /white wheat flour, salt and sugar , cooking fat/oil | Mix brown &white floor (1:1), salt and sugar to taste and knead the dough to desired quality. Cut pieces of dough and roll into flat circular sheets and place on the frying pan until brown, turn so that both sides are well cooked, add cooking fat or oil as desired. | 1 or 2 Chapatis used to be consumed before diagnosis but only half after diagnosis. |
| 3 | Peas Mukimo(Mash) | Green Peas, Green Maize, Irish Potatoes, Green Bananas Salt & water | Boil Green Peas and Green Maize until they are ready. Add Green whole peeled Green Bananas and Irish Potatoes and continue boiling until the last two are coked. Drain water and add salt to taste. Mix and Mash by twisting the flat wooden cooking spoon(muiko) that is used for that purpose | Choose Green Bananas that are sour(almost ripe) for a better taste |
| 5 | Black Beans (Njahi)Mukimo(Mash) | Black Beans, Ripe Bananas, Green Bananas, Irish Potatoes, Green Maize | Boil Black Beans and Green Maize until they are cooked. Add whole peeled Green Bananas and Irish Potatoes and continue boiling until they are cooked. Drain the water and return to the fire. Add one or two whole peeled ripe Bananas and cover for 1 to 2 minutes. Add salt to taste and mix as you Mash using a flat wooded spoon | Choose Green Bananas that are sour(almost ripe) for a better taste |
| | Greens Mukimo (Mash) | Consists of Green Maize, Green Pumpkin leaves( Kahurura), Irish Potatoes, | Boil Maize with or without Beans or Peas, when ready add whole peeled Potatoes and when the Potatoes are tender, add cleaned hand shred Green leaves and boil until they are cooked. Drain the water; add salt to taste and mix as you Mash to have a uniform consistency. Serve while hot. | |
| 6 | Apple, Cider Vinegar with Honey(ACVH) | Apple cider Vinegar, Honey, | Boil a glass of water, add a 5-10 mls of Apple cider vinegar and a table spoon of | Makes a tasty soothing drink  before retiring to bed |

| | | Water | honey; mix and take while hot | |
|---|---|---|---|---|
| 7 | Ndazi(one), Mandazi(many) | White wheat flour, Sugar, Salt, Baking Powder | Mandazi are similar to doughnuts but a bit puffy. Mix white wheat flour, sugar and baking powder. Add water and mix to make dough similar to that of Chapati. Roll the dough on a flat surface using a wooden round rod. Cut the flat dough into pieces of desired shapes, deep fry the pies in hot oil until brown. Serve while hot or cold. | The Mandazi normally have a high quantity of sugar that give them their characteristic taste. |
| 8 | Matumbo(Offals) | This could include a combination of liver, kidneys, heart, stomach and intestines of cattle, sheep or Goats | Clean the items thoroughly. As for the stomach and intestines, they are normally purchase from the butchery when all the food contents have professionally been expressed from them. Fry using cooking oil/fat. Add Tomatoes and other spices to taste. | The Goat Matumbo are tastier than the other maybe because they consume a variety of trees and shrubs while the other two consume grass most of the time. |
| 9 | Rice | Brown Rice | Boiled until cooked | Salt/ Margarine and or fats/oils that are included in boiling of Rice are excluded in this case. |
| 10 | RVM | Raw vegetable Mixed(RVM) | This is a salad made of a combination of locally and in season vegetables. Carrots, Cabbage, Onions and Tomatoes are almost always there. Others include pepper, Capsicum, parsley and cucumber among others. Salt, sugar, olive oil and other species could also be added | In this case, sugar, salt and spices were either minimal or excluded |
| 11 | Ugali | | **Ugali** (also sometimes called **Sima**, **Sembe** or **Posho**) is a dish of Maize flour (cornmeal). In this case, Ugali also had millet flour (wimbi), or Sorghum flour (Mtama), Any or a combination of the flours are added to boiling water and the flat wooden spoon is used to mix the flours while still on the fire  to produce a dough-like consistency. Mixing and mashing continue until a Sweet aroma, characteristic of the food comes out or until a firm crust covers the pot. Remove from the fire and serve while hot. | Cold Ugali is almost flat in taste. In this case Millet, sorghum and cassava flours used to be mixed at a ratio of 4:1:1 and the mixture preserved in a bowl and only small quantities used as required. This ensured an uniform mixture all the time |
| 12 | Oats bread | Whole wheat meal /Oats | Purchased ready-to-eat from a supermarket | Found in selected supermarkets |
| 14 | Nuts( Cashew nuts, Groundnuts, Almond nuts, Peanuts, Macadamia, and walnuts) | Nuts( Cashew nuts, Groundnuts, Almond nuts, Peanuts, Macadamia, and walnuts), Water, Salt | These were bought from the supermarkets as packaged ready to eat SNACKs prepared by  Roasting( pea, ground and Almonds) and steamed and dried (Cashew nuts) | These SNACKs either never consumed or consumed rarely and sparingly pre-diagnosis but became a common breakfast item post diagnosis. In most of the days that they were consumed, the GI was just slightly above 5, giving an indication that they might have some glycaemia reducing properties |
| 15 | Chicken Stew | Made from local birds | Unless otherwise stated refers to local free range Chicken fried with Onions and Tomatoes and water added to make at least a liter  of soup | |
| 16 | Deep fried Chicken | Made from broiler Chicken | Deep fry pieces of the meat in hot oil until brown or well cooked. Serve hot or cold | Sometimes the local Chicken could also be used, but on rare occasion |
| 17 | Local vegetables | cowpea leaves(Kunde), African nightshade leaves(Managu), Amaranthus (Terere) and others | Clean meticulously and boil. When tender drain the water and fry with Onions, Tomatoes and cooking oil/fat. Add salt to taste. Serve while hot. Use alone and or with foods like meat stews, Ugali, Matumbo and Mashed foods. | Best with Ugali |
| 18 | Samosa | White flour, Vegetables for vegetable Samosa | Prepare dough into a flat sheet as for Chapati. Cut the flat sheet in desired | Triangular shape gives the Samosa its characteristic |

| | | and minced meat for meat Samosas | shapes. In the middle of each piece, add well fried vegetables or minced meat. The food materials should contain as little water as possible. Roll over the edges of the piece of dough so as to cover the vegetable/ meat material. Deep fry in hot oil and serve while hot. | shape though it does not alter the taste. Spices in both meat or vegetable ingredients enhance the taste |
|---|---|---|---|---|
| 27 | Tubers | Arrow roots, Sweet Potatoes, Yams, cassava | Cleaned, boiled together with the peel, water drained when well cooked and served hot. Can be taken with tea or with any stew | Sweet Potatoes consumed with or without the peel while the core fibrous and suggestively poisonous part of cassava is removed |
| 28 | Omena(lake Victoria Sardine Fish) | Omena, Onions, Tomatoes, Lemon juice | Clean and rinse several times in hot water. Fry with Onions and cooking oil/fat. Add Tomatoes and Lemon juice and cook for 10-15 minutes. | Best with Ugali |
| 29 | Fish stew | Large size Tilapia(more than 500grams) , Onions, Tomatoes, Capsicum, parsley | Cut the Fish horizontally into two or more pieces depending on the size. Fry the Onions and Tomatoes together and add water enough to cover the Fish. When the mixture has boiled, put in the Fish. Continue cooking until the Fish has a firm consistency or the water level has gone down significantly. Serve while hot | This was a deviation from the pre-diagnosis stage when deep fried Fish was always consumed. It was one of the ways or reducing cholesterol and fats. |
| 30 | Toasted sandwich-Oats bread | Bread, Onions, Carrots | Grate a whole Carrots and a whole Onion. Apply Margarine a slice of bread on both sides, place it on a toaster, and cover it with the Carrots/Onion mixture. Apply Margarine on both sides of another slice of bread. Use it to cover the ingredients on the first slice. Cover the toasted, put on the heat and wait until it is brown in color. Take it hot with tea( **Annex 7)** | |
| 31 | Mursik | milk | Purchased lady Made but literature[19] indicate that it is made from cow or Goat milk and fermented in a specially made calabash ground. The gourd is lined with sooth from specific trees which add flavor to the fermented milk. It is normally consumed with Ugali or on its own and is served at room temperature or chilled. | |
| 32 | Maize & Beans(Githeri) | Maize, beans or peas | Boil a mixture of maize and beans. Drain water and add salt and consume alone or with tea.. You can also fry the mixture with oil and onions with or without additions such as vegetables or potatoes | |
| 33 | | | | |

Note: Some of the local names for the foods are in Kikuyu, Kiswahili or any of the languages of the over 40 tribes of Kenya

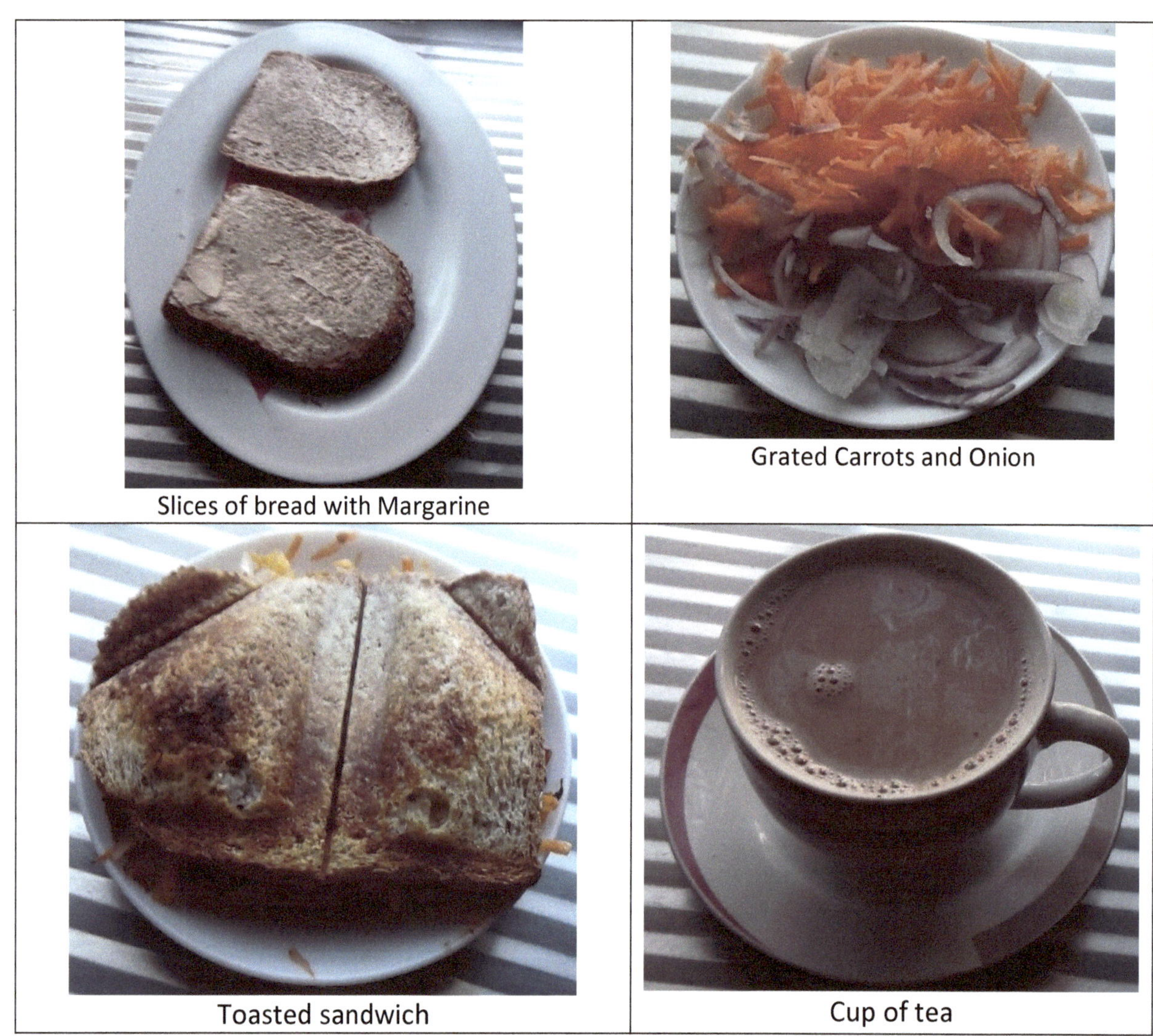

Slices of bread with Margarine

Grated Carrots and Onion

Toasted sandwich

Cup of tea

# REFERENCES

1. Duff, M., Demidova, O., Blackburn, S.& Shubrook, J.(2015). Cutaneous manifestations of diabetes mellitus. Clin Diabetes. 2015;33(1):40–48

2. Manson,J.E., Stampfer, M.J., Rosner, B.& Willett WC.(2002). Glycemic index, glycemic load, and risk of type 2 diabetes. Am J Clin Nutr 2002;76(suppl):274S–9S.

3. Riccardi, G., Rivellese, A.A. & Giacco, R.(2008). Role of glycemic index and glycemic load in the healthy state, ... and in diabetes. Am J Clin Nutr 2008;87(suppl):269S-74S

4. Elliott,P., Stamler,J., Nichols,R., Dyer,A.R., Stamler,R., Hugo Kesteloot,H., & Marmot, M.(1996). Intersalt revisited: further analyses of 24 hour sodium excretion and blood pressure within and across populations. *BMJ ;312:1249-53*

5. Furldell, E. L. (2009). *Fatal thirst: Diabetes in Britain until Insulin*. Leiden. Boston: *IDC* publishers, Martinus Nijhoff Publishers and vsp

6. Patient information; polycystic ovary syndrome. 2015 BMJ Group (2015). BMJ, p 1-4 Available http://besthealth-bmj.com/pdf/392705.pdf Accessed 12-04-2016

7. Taylor, R. (2013). Type 2 Diabetes: Etiology and reversibility. Diabetes Care, 36:1047-1055

8. University of IOWA Health Care (2016). Diabetic Ketoacidosis https://uihc.org/adam/1/diabetic-ketoacidosis Accessed 15-04-2016

9. Mayo clinic(1998-2016). Diseases and Conditions-Diabetic Neuropathy. http://www.mayoclinic.org/diseases-conditions/diabetic-neuropathy/basics/causes/con-20033336 accessed 13/8/2016

10. Gelabert, R. C. (2009). *A practical Guide to Health: Diabetes, Scientific and Natural Treatments.* Saragossa spain :Ediciones vidasana

11. Plat-McDonald, S.(2010). *How to add years to your life and life to your years: The little book of Health for seniors.* Grantham, Lincolnshire: The Stanborough Press Ltd

12. Burgess, A. & Glassauer, P.(2004). *Family nutrition guide*. Italy Rome: FAO

13. Min. of Agriculture & Min. of Public Health and sanitation (2013). Nairobi, Kenya: Applied basic Agri-Nutrition Resource Manual for trainees

14. WHO (2006). Definition and diagnosis of Diabetes Mellitus and intermediate hyperglycemia available *http://apps.who.int/iris/bitstream/10665/43588/1/9241594934_eng.pdf* Accessed 16-8-2016

15. Choi, K. M., Lee, J., Kim, D. R., Kim, S. K., Shin, D. H., Kim, N. H., Park, I. B., Choi, D. S. and Baik, S. H. (2002), Comparison of ADA and WHO criteria for the diagnosis of diabetes in elderly Koreans. Diabetic Medicine, 19: 853–857. doi: 10.1046/j.1464-5491.2002.00783.x

16. WHO (2013). A global brief on HYPERTENSION. Silent killer, global public health crises. Available http://ish-world.com/downloads/pdf/global_brief_hypertension.pdf Accessed 16-8-2016

17. Centers for disease control and prevention.(2015). Target Heart Rate and Estimated Maximum Heart Rate. Available

18. *https://www.cdc.gov/physicalactivity/basics/measuring/heartrate.htm* *Accessed 17-8-2016*

19. Njoki, C.( 2017, July 8).Health, family top list of what Kenyans care about most. *Saturday Nation, p.3.*

20. *Mursik.2017. Available* https://en.wikipedia.org/wiki/Mursik  Accessed 20-4-2017